Don't Eat Cancer

by Sean David Cohen

ⓒ Copyright 2014 by Sean David Cohen

ISBN 978-1-9401922-4-6

Published by

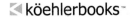 köehlerbooks™

210 6oth Street
Virginia Beach, VA 23451
212-574-7939
www.koehlerbooks.com

Publisher
John Köehler

Executive Editor
Joe Coccaro

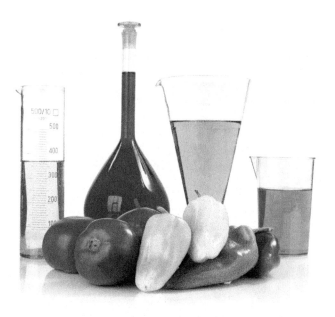

Also by Sean David Cohen

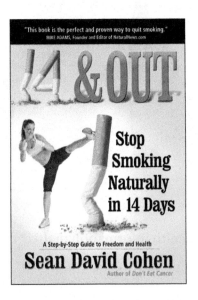

14 And Out—Stop Smoking Naturally in 14 Days!

Downloadable Video, DVD,
Paperback & E-Book

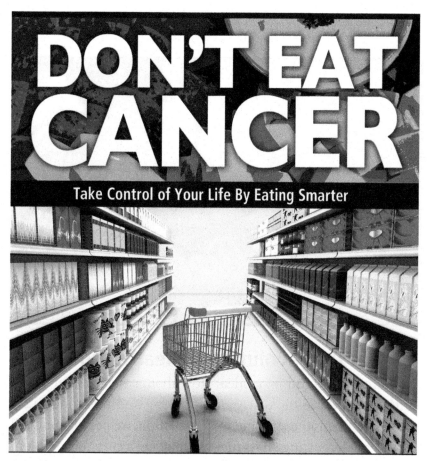

DON'T EAT CANCER

Take Control of Your Life By Eating Smarter

Sean David Cohen

Author of 14 & Out: Stop Smoking Naturally in 14 Days

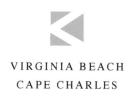

VIRGINIA BEACH
CAPE CHARLES

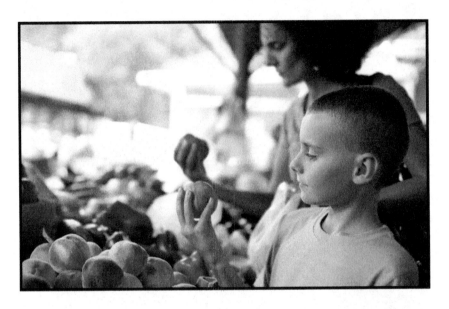

Join the revolution of healthy souls!

Here is a revolutionary idea: How about instead of surgically cutting out where the disease is attacking and then dousing it with toxic chemotherapy and toxic radiation, we prevent and kill the disease by cutting off its fuel—toxins! Let's cure this problem on the front end. It's time that you cut off the enemy supply lines by eliminating your intake of chemicals! Just as a general in the Army would do to weaken the front lines of the enemy, we give our body the ultimate fighting advantage.

Contents

Foreword

The great hidden truth of the for-profit cancer industry is that preventing cancer is remarkably easy. Most people wouldn't have cancer if they didn't give it to themselves; day after day, bite after bite, toxin after toxin.

While the cancer industry with all its pink ribbons and billions of dollars in funding pretends to be looking for a "cure" for cancer, it utterly neglects to acknowledge the far simpler answer found in day-to-day prevention. The cure for cancer, it turns out, must begin with an honest discussion about what causes cancer. And that's a discussion in which the cancer industry absolutely refuses to engage.

Why? Because if you talk honestly about the causes of cancer, you just might stumble upon a way to slash cancer rates by 50, 60 or even 90 percent. Those of us who actually do focus on cancer prevention know that cancer is a disease that people, for the most part, unknowingly give to themselves.

With each bite of processed meat that's laced with sodium nitrite—and that's a common ingredient in hot dogs, sausage, bacon, jerkies and sandwich meat—we are increasing our risk for colon cancer, pancreatic cancer and brain tumors. Every bite of an apple pie with a crust made with hydrogenated oils also adds to our cancer risk, and recent research at the Natural News Forensic Food Lab shows that even many superfoods, vegan protein products and USDA organic food products contain very concerning concentrations of the heavy metal arsenic, a toxic substance known to contribute to cancer risk.

Eating cancer is so common across the American culture, that fast food, cancer centers and runaway medical costs have become routine ... even "normalized." The personal pursuit of food-based "slow suicide" via processed foods and junk foods laced with cancer-causing chemicals is so commonplace in our culture that nearly all thoughts of potential links between food and cancer have been lost to history. Just because suicidal behaviors become socially acceptable doesn't mean they are any less harmful, however. The American pastime of pizza, donuts, fast food and artificial food is precisely what is killing our brothers and sisters, mothers and fathers, and even children and infants whose lives could be saved at very little economic cost by simply choosing foods which prevent cancer instead of causing it.

It took the medical establishment over five decades to finally realize that smoking causes cancer. The days of the Journal of the American Medical Association running full-page ads for Camels cigarettes are long gone, of course, but the organization really did earn tremendous profits from selling cancer to its own readers and followers. How long will it take for the medical establishment to admit that today's popular foods also contain cancer-causing substances which contribute to millions of deaths each year? Probably another five decades if history teaches us anything.

Until the medical establishment comes to its senses on the causal relationships between food choice and cancer risk, you'll need to turn to informed educators who are ahead of the curve—people like Sean David Cohen and this book, *Don't Eat Cancer*. Here's where you will find the answers that modern medicine won't admit for another few decades.

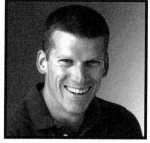

By that time, of course, tens of millions of other people will have died from a disease which is almost 100% preventable by those who have the right information. This book gives you that information in a concise, easy-to-read format that I know can not only inspire millions of people to live healthier lives, it can also contribute to quite literally saving millions of lives for years to come.

"Don't eat cancer" is very good advice and a motto to live by.

—Mike Adams, Food Research Director, Natural News
Forensic Food Labs, Editor, NaturalNews.com

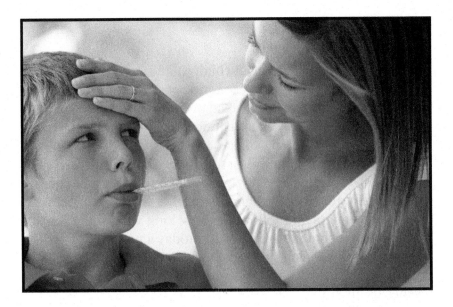

When I was a kid, if I got a migraine headache or a stomach ache, or I was lethargic all day, my mother always asked me what I ate over the past twenty four hours. She would make me go through every drink and every morsel of food, until she figured it out. *She almost always blamed the food for our small, but chronic, health problems.* After interrogating my sisters and me about what we ate, she usually discovered the source of our ailments.

I decided not to let my mother's wisdom go to waste. One day I had so much useful information in my head about the common chemicals in foods and all the food agents, I decided to write a book. I had already written two fiction novels, but this was different.

Now I had a chance to help millions of people with all of the information I had stored in my head, and all the things my mother and I had researched. It was time to get it all on paper. But cancer is not an easy subject to understand or communicate to others. I used my journalism degree from the University of Georgia to propel my writing and publishing efforts. Also, in the late 90's, I was a fifth grade school teacher in Athens,

Georgia. I taught all subjects to the same 23 kids all day. One thing I learned from that experience was to have patience with my delivery of information. Sometimes, if something was really important, I would have to teach the same strategy, idea or concept five different ways in fifteen- to-thirty-minute increments so they would all understand.

My approach to sharing knowledge about cancer and cancer prevention is similar. I want to make sure you understand WHAT cancer is, HOW it works against your cells, WHERE it comes from, and WHEN it spreads, so that you know exactly how to cut off its fuel. When you cut off cancer's fuel, you cut the head off the snake. This is a war you can win.

Some people feel overwhelmed by all the health information out there, in books, in the news, on television, and in magazines. They don't know what to believe and it's just all too complicated. This is exactly what makes *Don't Eat Cancer* unique. It is written in laymen's terms for ordinary people. I am neither a doctor nor a licensed medical expert of any kind. *The science of cancer is complicated and anyone with the disease or with symptoms of it should be guided by a licensed medical professional.*

I also don't mean to be insensitive to those who are ill with the disease or who have lost a loved one to cancer. This book is not about assigning blame, it's about punching holes in myths about how and why cancer is so widespread and empowering individuals with the knowledge that they can take steps—simple steps—to decrease the risks of contracting cancer, avoiding it altogether and, possibly, fighting it off once it invades their body.

There is no doubt that some in the scientific community, and almost certainly advocates for chemical makers, will dispute or dismiss some of what is alleged in these pages. They'll argue the chemicals infused in our foods are "proven" safe and that they're closely regulated and must meet the highest levels of safety testing. They'll evoke study-after-study proving their point. My point is that while any individual product may, in fact, have "safe" levels of some poison, no one is measuring the cumulative effect of the sea of preservatives, additives and other junk in *all* of what we eat. You cannot gauge the safety of our food bite by bite. Since the federal regulators don't look at the cumulative effect of chemicals in our food, you, as a consumer, must. Don't rely on the food industry to protect you; protect yourself.

What I am offering as a trained observer and researcher is making very complicated science easy to understand. I avoid some medical terminology and jargon nobody can understand, or at least not enough to take action and filter their daily diet. You see, it is my belief that cancer is a cumulative effect of toxins in the body, and by eliminating your daily intake of toxins linked to cancer you reduce the risk of contracting some form of the disease. ***This book helps you avoid the toxins by teaching you where they exist in the foods we eat.*** Learning this information is what I call the basement of basics. It's not just simple to understand, it is super simple. People make it too complicated, but *Don't Eat Cancer* breaks it all down for you. Here are some of the facts this book is based upon, and the alarming statistics I aim to lower by sharing the strategies that allow you to cut off the fuel that feeds the fire.

In the United States alone, cancer attacks every other man and every third

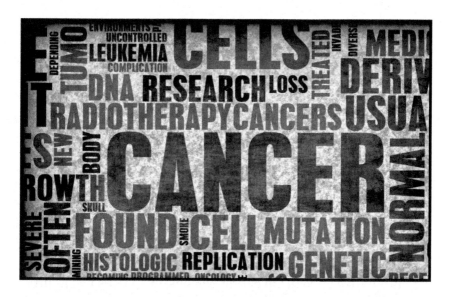

woman. There is generally a fifty percent survival rate. That means your chances of contracting cancer at some point in your life are high. You need a plan to improve those odds. You can't sit around playing a guessing game with what you eat, drink, and put on your skin. In this case, what you don't know will hurt you. You need to know what chemicals the FDA is allowing in your food, what the latest names for them are, and how they can affect your immune system and your vitality. Make informed decisions. There is a cumulative effect from consuming just a little bit of toxins every day.

There are more than seventy thousand chemical agents allowed in our food supply that cause your cells to mutate, divide and multiply. You don't have to be a victim! Understand what cancer is, where it comes from, and how to impede its development. This user friendly guide reveals chemicals in products many people have never even considered. Sharing of this simple yet crucial information about chemicals in foods stems from my passion for mass communication. I want this message to reach millions of consumers, in every country of the world.

Once you read *Don't Eat Cancer* you're better prepared to protect yourself instead of relying on complex mathematical formulas used by federal regulators and chemical makers to estimate safe levels of ingestible toxins. This book will teach you—at the very least—the right questions to ask and facts to consider. Your entire purchasing regimen will change for good and you will feel much better. You will understand all about GMO or "GM" (genetically modified food), gluten and other toxic food additives. Each chapter is focused on a major area of concern regarding food, drinks, candy and gum, artificial sweeteners, personal care products, cigarettes and cosmetics. You learn exactly how cells mutate after consuming too many "agents" and how you can reverse that process by filtering them all out of your daily intake.

One central point of this book and my research is that there is a cumulative effect from eating poisons, even if it's just a "little bit" each day. That's what people forget to think about. It's dangerous to consider any one chemical in a vacuum. The point I'll make over and over in this book is that *we must consider the cumulative effect of the sea of toxins washing into our bodies each day.* Just as you have to be a defensive driver to avoid accidents, you have to be a defensive consumer to avoid all of the chemicals that you can ingest on a daily basis. *Don't Eat Cancer* is like your drivers education course for avoiding chemicals that can kill you. This modern approach is simple yet so comprehensive. Learn how to be your own body guard. Put guards at the gates of your temple (your body and soul). Don't let cancer in. *Don't Eat Cancer* and it won't eat you. Remember, knowledge means power, so I invite you to join me in this quest for longevity. These simple, preventive revelations are better than a thousand surgeons' knives and more effective than gallons of chemotherapy after it's already too late.

Change the way you look at the cure for cancer. View it as a disciplined, active prevention plan, and the cure will follow. Even if you already have cancer, if you stop pouring in the poisons, your good cells will have a much better chance of fighting and surviving the bad ones. If you were getting sick from moldy bread, would you look for a cure from a vaccine, or medicine, or consider surgery, while you keep on eating more moldy bread every day?

There are thousands of libraries and bookstores filled with hundreds of thousands of books telling you what to eat to stay healthy and hopefully live a long, fruitful life. But most of the time, it's not what we choose to eat that matters so much, it's what we don't filter out of food that makes the difference.

Start thinking about what not to eat. About-face your thinking. And realize it's not your fault that you've been fooled. Big corporations still legally camouflage chemicals and toxins they use to produce our foods—to make them bigger, prettier, meatier, and of course, tastier. It's not so much that corporations want to kill us, they just don't care. It's all about the money. If some chemical is going to improve the overall marketability and sales of a product, or produce twice as many for less, then they simply payoff the politicians or regulators who would normally restrict and/or ban those chemicals from being approved, and those people "sell out", and we the consumers pay the ultimate price with our lives.

Cut out your bad habits by reading the labels and setting the chemicals back on the shelf. They'll stop selling. The cure is in our hands, when we stop ourselves and think—between when we look at the ingredients on the back of the box, and when we buy it, cook it and put it in our mouths, or on our skin. The cure is not feeding disease more poison. *The cure is not poisoning already poisoned cells.* Then the healthy cells can do their job. It's like the war on terror. It doesn't start on the battlefield; it starts in the schools, through education.

In the same light, beating cancer starts with identifying and then eliminating the chemicals we use and eat on a regular basis, because it is enough to kill us, and it does kill us in a host of diseases we call cancer. Stop thinking only about what to eat, and learn WHAT NOT TO EAT!

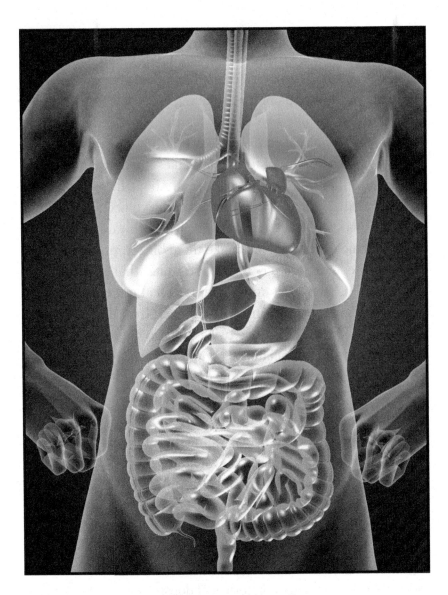

Chapter 1
Guards at the Gates

Corporations are like spiders that weave webs of poison in food, drinks, candy, gum, baby formula and lotions. Cancer's army of webs attacks the unknowing and the weak. Among children ages fourteen and under , cancer causes more deaths in the U.S. than any other disease. Big corporations use chemicals and by-products (obvious carcinogens) that they know are dangerous because it makes them more money. It preserves their products longer or makes them look and taste better. Food company advocates argue that preservatives and other chemicals makes food safer because it won't spoil and it makes it more affordable because of less waste. Maybe so. Maybe it translates to lower costs at the supermarket. But what is the real cost? Your health, medical bills, feeling bad. Food manufacturers put your health on the shelf, as it's directly heading for the ultimate, incurable disease, and we just seem to ignore it all until it's too late. **In this case, ignorance is not bliss, its death by cancer.**

The average life expectancy of humans right now is age seventy three. Cancer will kill sixteen percent of those people before that age; many will be children. *Cancer will kill more than seven hundred and fifty thousand people this year.* That's one hundred Super Bowl stadiums full of people—gone forever.

Okay then, let's talk about what causes this epidemic. Carcinogens directly cause cancer. Have no doubts about it. They are chemical agents and compounds that impair cellular respiration. Your cells need oxygen to breath just like your lungs. Oxygen deficiency at the cellular level breeds cancer.

Cancer is the uncontrolled alteration and division of specific cells, and the ability of those cells to invade and corrode other body tissues.

Chemicals or physical "agents" called carcinogens enter our bodies, causing unnatural cell divisions and cell mutations that turn and attack our already weakened, damaged, or predisposed tissue.

Your organs are like a moth caught in a spider web, and just as a spider senses when its prey is vulnerable, so do the chemically altered cell mutations that turn and attack any weakened tissue. On X-rays, most cancer looks just like spider webs. Have you ever seen an X-ray of cancer at the latent stages, when it invades organs and chokes them out? It looks a lot like when a spider cocoons a bug, but in humans it's your organs that get cocooned.

Understand that it's very hard to stop cancer once it develops in your system, because damaged cells and tissues in your body are very susceptible to warped cells that begin pitching their webs in the blood—webs that are basically fueled by the chemicals you and I pour into our systems on a daily basis.

If you don't learn the names of all the poisons, and you just stick to your old ways and continue eating fake sugars and microwaving your food, then the newly mutated cells will join up with the older "bad guys" and travel through your body, searching for a host organ that's weak, or a spot of skin that's been burned over and over by the sun, or maybe a lung that's been "smoked out" for twenty years, and take it over.

For many smokers, but not all, cancer spreads like spider webs in the lungs, suffocating its victims to death. For women, sometimes the mutated gang goes after a breast, because that breast has a small tumor developing from the abnormal influx of growth hormones that came from the chickens and pigs and cows consumed, animals that had been shot up with steroids for years before they were slaughtered, prepped, and rushed to your favorite fast food joints. All of that meat helps give us cancer, and still we keep eating it, because it's hot, cheap, fast, and sometimes tastes good. ***Nobody said healthy was easy, if it*** *was, everyone would live to be one hundred.*

Ever heard of someone having cancer and the doctors go in and do invasive surgery and then tell the patient, "Go home buddy. We got it!"

Then a few months later it creeps up somewhere else in the body, and the person is devastated by the news. I've heard of it. I hear it a lot. It's very sad. At the least the doctors should warn patients of their chances of relapse, and guide them with proper diet and "chemical avoidance" advice.

I know more than a few people to whom this has happened, but we keep pouring in the chemicals! They even serve *artificial sweeteners* in hospitals. "Hey, doctors and nurses trying to heal me, I'll have an iced tea without *rat poison*, please, and make it a rush! While you're at it, bring me some processed GMO food with gluten from the hospital cafeteria. Oh, and bring me a clipboard and a pen, I have some questions for you people running this place."

Big questions for the medical industry: Could it be that the operation to *remove* the cancer was in fact a mission just to extract the tissue that the web was attacking? What about when some of the web gets away while under the knife?

Isn't that why the victims of this chemically induced disease get called back in when they find out some "got away", or in other words, the web moved? Let me tell you the truth now.

Filtering most chemicals from your product selection at the store is your main chance for long term survival. It's easy; just do it. Instead of just cutting out where the disease is attacking, we kill the disease by cutting off its fuel just like generals in a war cutting off an enemy's supply line. But we don't do that. Our medical industry is based on treating the problem after it exists and persists, after it's a chronic issue.

Are we still cavemen? Why do so many people ignore the

common sense approach to cancer prevention? Take a deep breath now and contemplate this notion: If you have a problem with weeds growing in the back yard, do you just walk around with clippers to remove the tops of them, thinking they'll go away? Is that the cure? No.

You have to dig for the roots. *Cancer has roots, and those roots feed off of the chemicals we eat, drink and put on our skin.* Stop feeding the weeds. Choose to start a healthier lifestyle right now. Consider this *Chemical Treatment Warning*: Damage done by an unsuccessful course of chemo is so bad that one's immune system sometimes never recovers. Be your own researcher and find a cancer specialist that uses a state-of-the-art chemotherapy program that's been proven successful in a good percentage of cases. Imagine having no immune system, that's like the final stages of AIDS or kidney failure. Start filtering more chemicals out of your diet now, or the future could be grim.

Allow me to get political for a moment. Do not donate money to cancer funds that just look for a cure on the back end of the problem. Fund preventative medicine. And when you do give make sure most of the money goes for science and research, not administrative costs. We should start spending more cancer research money on regulations for keeping chemicals out of our foods and body lotions, instead of surgically cutting them out of our bodies after the fact.

Our typical grocery store has toxins in three out of every four items on the shelf, and there's no stopping all of these big corporations from producing them, and there's no stopping the FDA from releasing them, while they settle lawsuits with about one-thousandth of the profits.

Meanwhile, the temples of our souls are slowly taken over, and our major organs suffocated, until we die an ugly, untimely death, earlier than we ever anticipated.

Cancer is like a fire: cut off the fuel first, and then you can snuff out the rest. Just like when a fire reaches a fuel supply, most cancers spread through the lymph, the clear fluid that bathes body cells. That's cancer's outlet. It uses the lymph nodes like catapults, traveling in the blood to spread new cancers in other parts of the body.

The medical community has it wrong, for the most part. They're running us in a big, useless circle. It's a vicious cycle so they can keep making money. Cancer is not a disease. It's a mutation of your cells that gang up and attack your own body. That's not the same thing as disease. It's a civil war inside your body, and as long as you eat chemicals, the bad guys get stronger, and eventually, they take your life. *All you have to do to help your own body beat cancer is to stop eating chemicals, and stop putting them on your body.* That's the cure for what they call disease. Read the labels; know the killers. Most importantly, put guards at the gates!

Fast food is the ultimate killer because it sneaks in under our radar, because it's so cheap, hot, fast, and tasty. Why does it suck the life out of us? That's obvious—cheese and butter. Think about just a few of the cancers out there for a second: lung cancer, skin cancer, intestinal cancer, prostate cancer, breast cancer, cancer of the liver, cancer of the kidneys, cancer of the stomach, and the list just goes on and on. Corporate America has become like an undercover terrorist, invading us when we think all is safe, except in this case the enemy gets paid a lot more money to do it ... However, there is a pot of gold at the end of the rainbow called good health.

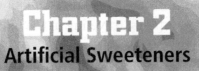

Chapter 2
Artificial Sweeteners

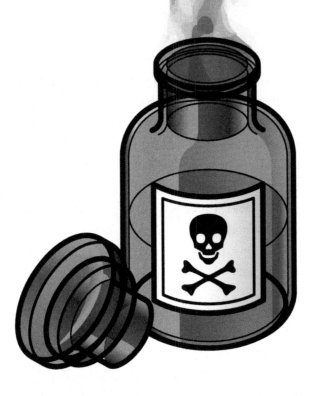

Stand in any grocery store line and look to your right and left. Every sugar free candy or gum, except for chocolate, is pumped full of chemicals. Pick up any one of them and flip it over and read the ingredients and you'll find at least one of the following: *Sorbitol, Sucralose, Saccharin, Equal, Splenda, Nutrasweet, BHT, Acesulfame, Aspartame,* or *Spoonful.* The breath mints, the gum, the sugar free gum, you name it and there's a boatload of chemicals in them. And if it's the first item on the list of ingredients, then guess what, that means there's more of that than any other ingredient! Yep, nice little cancer pills for you and me to suck on for fresh breath, and hey, "without the calories!"

Rule of thumb: If it tastes sweet, and it's not sweetened naturally, then chances are there's a chemical in it doing the job. It'll do a job on you too! Call it a *final extraction.* Plus, now they're putting Sucralose, Aspartame and Acesulfame-K in candy that isn't even a sugar-free item. Why? These additives are used as softeners to keep gum soft for longer shelf life. You better start reading the ingredients on everything. You may also want to check your toothpaste, your mouthwash, your contact lens solution, your diet drinks, and yes, even check your chewable multivitamin, especially some of the flavored kids brands. Believe it or not, they're loaded with chemical sweetness. And I mean loaded. Read the ingredients. What you don't know can hurt you. Do more research. Go organic. Check out the Natural News website for a list of good ones:

http://www.naturalnews.com/033702_chemicals_vitamins.html

There's an invasion of chemicals in vitamins and supplements. Synthetic vitamins fuel sickness while enriching the corrupt medical industry. Could you be taking a multi-vitamin that's killing you slowly? Check it out:

http://www.naturalnews.com/036650_synthetic_vitamins_disease_side_effects.html

Can you imagine, you're sitting there taking multivitamins to improve your health, and they're contaminated with some of the same stuff that kills rats—*sorbitol, saccharin, aspartame, equal, nutrasweet, sucralose, splenda.* The list includes fancy brand names that sound like a normal natural ingredient, to brand names you thought were product names. Some of the chemicals in them give rats tumors and cancer.

And I know what you're thinking now, but you're wrong. Don't think for a second we're not composed like those little varmints they test in the labs, because we are.

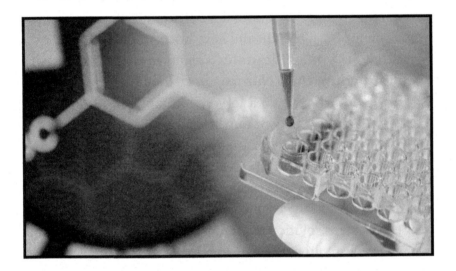

The Ninety-Nine Percent Rule

Humans have ninety-nine percent the same genetic makeup of DNA as the mice and rats tested in labs. Though most of us do not scavenge in dumpsters, sifting through rotten food for our dinner, our bodies are affected by chemical food all the same. This is where people underestimate the impact of scientific studies done on rats. Think about it, artificial sugars are just that, they are fake and cause horrible health side effects, including seizures and tumors. Imitation sugars are chemical agents, like double agents, and they fool the body into ingesting them because the body senses they are sweet. That's the big killer. Your body would normally work hard to get rid of these poisons, but the sweet taste tricks it. *Your organs get fooled and fail to filter out the toxins.* Research shows some of the agents used never leave the body, but build up residually in the cleansing organs, like the liver, the kidneys, and the pancreas. Your kidneys, your liver, your spleen, your gall bladder, your stomach, your intestines, and many other vital organs can't do their job if they can't recognize poison, so don't let your guard down. Rule all imitation sugars out of your diet, now.

Current statistics show there were one million four hundred thousand million people in the U.S. diagnosed with cancer in 2006, and half of those people died. They died! Yet, the experts always say the same thing, "There's not enough of the chemical agent in the food to cause a human being to develop cancer." How many times have we heard that? Well, that may be true of any one product, but add it up with the other fifty to sixty chemicals we consume everyday—day after day, and year after year—and it is enough to do serious damage.

The proof is in the pudding, and the pudding is poison. We are eating chemicals and they're killing us. How else can it be told? How else can you cure cancer?! Imagine, people who are actually fighting cancer are eating and drinking chemicals, like diet drinks, and they do it every day, all while they are "hoping" to heal.

Sucralose and Sorbitol

What are Sucralose and Sorbitol? How do companies make them, and where do they come from? Sucralose is the tricky one, because Sucralose sounds just like sucrose. While sucrose is another name for natural sugar -watch out friends, sucralose is an artificial sweetener known by the trade name Splenda, which is a chemical substance and not a natural sugar. And, since money rules over health when it comes to our government, the CDC and the FDA, we've seen a repeat of the aspartame approval process for sucralose and sorbitol, allowing products with proven carcinogens to invade and flood our food, candy, gum, medicine, toothpaste and mouthwash supply.

The cure: *Eat brown sugar, raw sugar or honey instead.* Even white sugar is bleached, so steer clear of that. The only sugar substitutes I find now that are safe are natural herb-based products made from stevia and xylitol.

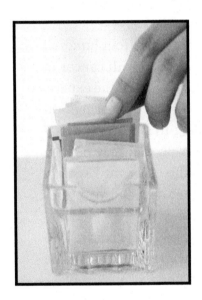

Aspartame—the King of Toxins

Aspartame is the worst of the fake sugar concoctions, without a doubt. Aspartame is a by-product of e-coli. It wrecks the central nervous system slowly and methodically. People highly underestimate the power of this synthetic lab concoction. Did you know seventy five percent of all complaints the FDA receives each year have to do with aspartame. Thousands of people have websites and letters of complaint posted swearing that this *additive* turns into poison in your system. It converts to formaldehyde in your body, which then turns into formic acid—the poison found in the sting of fire ants. Symptoms of multiple sclerosis and systemic lupus are very similar to the side effects of this sweet poison.

Here is more of what happens to your system when it takes in aspartame and other artificial sweeteners daily: Shrunken thymus glands, enlarged liver and kidneys, atrophy of lymph follicles in the spleen and thymus, reduced growth rate, decreased red blood cell count (that's what AIDS does to people), hyperplasia of the pelvis, special for the females is extension of the pregnancy period, aborted pregnancy, decreased fetal body weights and placental weights, and of course, the ever popular— diarrhea. Yippee! You may also have excessive shedding of hair or impact your liver's functioning. Add depression, anxiety and headaches to the list. Not good! Stop drinking diet drinks and eating sugar-free candy and gum—they are loaded. I actually found sucralose in whole wheat English muffins the other day. Come on!

Sucralose Breaks Down into a Chemical

Despite the manufacturer's misstatements, sucralose does break down into small amounts of dichloro-fructose, a chemical that has not been adequately tested on humans. Oh, but by the way, the *other* animals being tested are actually dying. Also don't forget that humans are animals. As for sorbitol, check this out: Corporations put sorbitol in contact lens solution. Opti-Free still has it. That's that new *softener* they're all adding. Can you imagine, we're putting this chemical right into our eyes! Maybe I should just use gasoline to clean my contact lenses, and then I'll "soften them up" with some baby oil. Are kids using this chemical too? I'm sure they are. I got contact lenses when I was twelve years old. Glad they didn't make sorbitol then! Tell your kids, if you still have them. Also, additive/preservatives BHA & BHT are totally unnecessary. These two closely related chemicals are added to oil-containing foods to prevent oxidation and slow rancidity. California has listed them as carcinogens. Let's all wake up and smell the coffee.

Acesulfame-K (Acesulfame Potassium)

They make it sound so safe, like it's just potassium or something, but beware! This killer additive is inadequately tested. The additive caused cancer in animals, which means it may increase cancer risk in humans. In 1987, CSPI (Center for Science in the

Public Interest) urged the FDA not to approve acesulfame, but was ignored. Is acesulfame potassium in your protein shake? Is this synthetic funk, also known as acesulfame-K, in your chewing gum? What is this stuff really made from and what does it do to your body? Is it just like aspartame, a known cancer causing and genetically modified sweetener? Does it mess with your central nervous system, sending you to some quack doctor for medicine to calm your nerves? Does it stay in your cleansing organs and in your small and large intestines for long periods of time, wreaking havoc on your digestive process and your whole excretive system?

How many people are eating and drinking products that contain this food toxin? How long has it been legalized for consumption and why doesn't the FDA regulate or ban it altogether? Just how many tens of thousands of people are writing letters to the food regulators about this artificial food category better known as *sweet misery*?

(http://www.youtube.com)

Acesulfame-K (aka "Ace-K") is a potassium salt containing methylene chloride, a known carcinogen. Acesulfame-K is not the same thing as aspartame, but quite often, both are found in the same products. Reported side effects of *sweet devil* acesulfame-K are frightening: "Long term exposure to methylene chloride can cause nausea, headaches, mood problems, impairment of the liver and kidneys, problems with eyesight and possibly cancer. Acesulfame-K may contribute to hypoglycemia."

http://www.fitday.com

Also, of all the artificial sweeteners out there, acesulfame-K has undergone the least scientific scrutiny. Early studies showed a link to multiple cancer developments in lab animals. If you have any doubts whatsoever, remember this; humans have ninety-nine percent the same DNA as the lab mice and rats tested. The proof is in the pudding! The research is concrete.

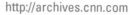

http://archives.cnn.com

This carcinogen, so cutely nicknamed Ace-K, is derived from aceto-acetic acid and fluoro-sulfonyl iso-cyanate. Say that last part again and it sounds like you're eating cyanide. Consider your total health risks before consuming ANY artificial sweetener.

http://www.naturalnews.com/041510_Ace-sulfame-K_methylene_chloride_carcinogen.html#ixzz2bh2vFulh

Of course we can't filter out every single by- product they slip into our foods, but we can catch most of them. The goal is to catch most of them. However, *if you know the chemicals are there, and you still consume them daily, well, that's just negligence.* For example, if you leave the toilet lid up, and your dog or cat drinks water out of it, and the toilet water has that blue stuff with hazardous cleansers like bleach in it, then you may know why your pet gets leukemia later on in life. There is an evil mutation of cells going on under our noses, and the numbers are sneaking up on us all.

War on Food

Welcome to the *Food War* my friends, you can fight or lose, it's your choice! And why is that a choice? Because there's no ignoring this war, and that's a cold fact that's hard to digest. Remember, the FDA and chemical by-product companies can't run these chemical tests on humans because that's considered inhumane. And it is. So, all the corporations justify their chemicals as being safe solely on the fact that, *"We aren't lab rats, and we might not be affected like those little animals."* We are, we just don't dig in dumpsters or drink out of the toilet, well, not most of us at least. Instead, we go shopping in stores with our credit cards to spend money like blind clones living and dying off their chemicalized products. Here's some simple rules of discipline: Remember, if it tastes sweet, usually too sweet, and the label says "sugar free", "light" or "zero", you have to check the ingredients for rat poison. They love hiding the poison in products that say *light*. Popular brands of ice cream and diet drink mixes serve it up like candy.

For almost all fake sugars, independent studies prove that they cause the rapid and uncontrolled growth of aberrant cells that will turn into malignant tumors over time. One of the worst is saccharin. And remember, the earlier in the list the ingredient is listed, the more of it that's in there. Saccharin is three hundred and fifty times sweeter than sugar. Animal studies have shown that it causes cancer of the bladder, uterus, ovaries, skin, blood vessels, and other organs. It also increases the potency of other cancer-causing chemicals, in other words, it's abetting other chemical criminals. There are new names for these serial killers every season. Now I see they call them *Sweet Plus, Splenda, Indulge, and Splenda Essentials*. We all have to keep up or we'll be "knocked down".

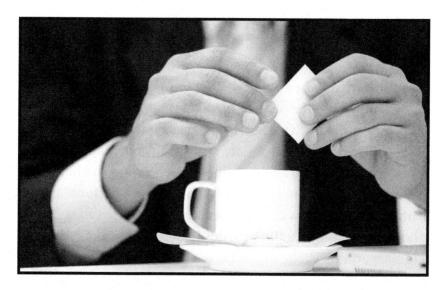

Artificial Sweetener Disease

Artificial Sweetener Disease (ASD) is sweeping across America, affecting tens of thousands of consumers, and Western medicine calls it anything but what it really is, so that doctors can prescribe expensive pharmaceuticals and set up "check up" appointments for the following weeks.

Call it recurring headaches, unbearable migraines, depression, anxiety, muscle pain, arthritis flare ups, buzzing or ringing in the ears, chronic fatigue, fibromyalgia, irritable bowel syndrome (IBS), Crohn's disease, inflammation, even acid reflux, but don't call it ASD, or the patient may stop consuming synthetic sweeteners, and then not schedule more doctor visits.

The symptoms of ASD can change overnight, depending on how much chemical sweetener you consume, and which ones. Some combinations are especially toxic. ***Consumers can go from a migraine headache to vomiting, or from vision problems to an upset stomach.*** Many people experience central nervous system disorders, cramping, nervous twitches and abnormal reflexes.

http://www.holisticmed.com/aspartame/

Learn more online:

http://www.naturalnews.com/034378_artificial_sweetener_disease_ASD_as-partame.html#ixzz2baRCdVSo

It all started when Ronald Reagan took office in 1980. He immediately fired the head of the FDA, under advisement from Donald Rumsfeld,CEO of Searle Pharmaceutical at the time, and hired Dr. Arthur Hull Hayes, Jr., who auspiciously approved aspartame. It was the decade of the diet craze, and the infamous Donald Rumsfeld and his constituents made a fortune off the artificial sweetener, which had been banned for decades due to laboratory testing results proving it was carcinogenic. Rumsfeld's aspartame is one of the biggest food blights on mankind. The same FDA tainted approval process gave way to sucralose in 1991, and then sorbitol in 2003.

Big corporations are about making big money; they're about selling products, not making people live better. Argue with me all you want, but numbers don't lie.

The top ten U.S. pharmaceutical companies spend eighty five percent of their money on advertising to sell us stuff, and only about fifteen on research and safety testing. The CEO's of these companies rank in the top fifty highest-paid persons in the country, averaging as a group fifteen billion a year, with up to five times that figure in stock options. Think about that for a minute. Who's profiting off your sickness?

In April 2000, Pharmacia & Upjohn completed a merger with Monsanto and Searle—creating a monstrous Pharmacia. In August 2002, Pharmacia completed the spin-off of its agricultural subsidiary, Monsanto Company. Pfizer and Pharmacia Corporations began operating as a unified company in 2003, forging the world's most powerful toxic-medicine-creating and distributing giant ever.

No prescription in existence cures ASD

There is no prescription drug, and there never will be one, that cures the problems that artificial sweeteners create. In fact, over seventy percent of reported cases of fibromyalgia, chronic depression, IBS and acid reflux are caused by consuming chemical agents, which have been approved by the FDA for consumption. Cancer may be the distant, long term result of consuming chemicals, but ASD is the short-term consequence, and it is very serious. If you look to prescription drugs to cure these chronic ailments, then you will experience even more side effects from the prescription medicines, and maybe worse ones than you already have.

The good news is the cure for *Artificial Sweetener Disease* is absolutely free and involves no doctors, no health insurance co-pays, and has zero side effects. Here is the secret cure for ASD: throw away your sugar free gum and candy, and then trash all foods and drinks you have that are labeled "light" and "zero." Read the labels on everything, so you can filter out all artificial sweeteners from your products, including aspartame, sucralose, sorbitol, acesulfame-k, aspartic acid, and saccharine.

Professional Articles/Research

http://www.foodintol.com/food_intolerance/irritable_bowel_syndrome

http://www.holisticmed.com/aspartame/

http://www.huffingtonpost.com/robbie-gennet/donald-rumsfeld-and-the-s...

http://www.militaryspot.com/resources/gulf_war_syndrome/

http://www.aspartamekills.com/mpvalley/

http://www.medicinenet.com/artificial_sweeteners/page8.htm

http://www.earthclinic.com/CURES/aspartame.html

http://www.foodintol.com/food_intolerance/irritable_bowel_syndrome

http://healthwyze.org/index.php/component/content/article/383-why-a-s...

http://www.thepanelist.net/general-finance-10103/1231-orbit-gum-white...

http://www.naturalnews.com/034320_aspartame_sweetener_side_effects.ht...

http://www.naturalnews.com/033914_Splenda_Essentials_sweetener.html

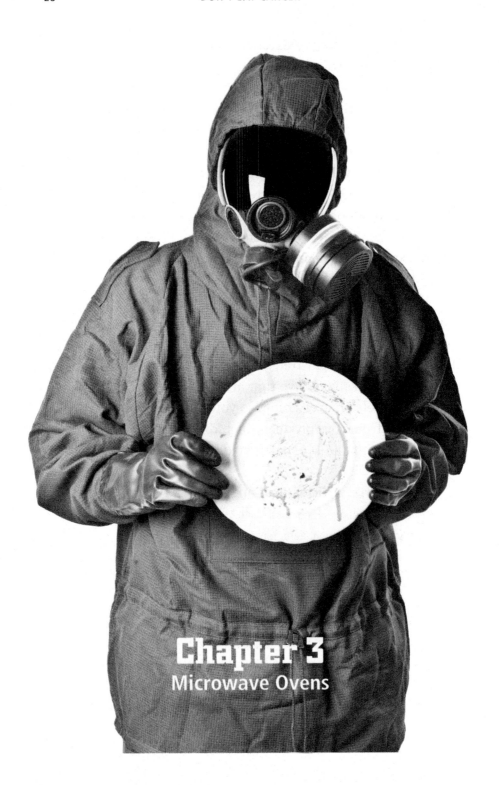

Chapter 3
Microwave Ovens

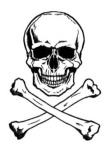 There's a reason we call them *Nukers*—they kill us! Put quite simply, you are radiating your food. The water molecules in the food are agitated at such a volatile pace that it destroys any nutrition and warps the structure of the food. That is what creates the heat. Ever notice they put a lead blanket over your vital, reproductive organs when you get x-rayed? That's to save you from the *cancer* rays. ***So why then would you put your food through a similar process that mutates it, and then eat it?*** I wonder why *convenience* so easily wins the war over good health. As a human race, we should realize that the latest simple conveniences welcome with them actual biological effects on your system, and these effects are doing damage in the temple of your soul. These biological effects include degeneration within the medulla oblongata, the frontal lobe of your brain that separates us from all the other non-planning, non-philosophical types of animals. You also get with that platter of health a long-term cumulative energy loss, with a gradual breakdown of the digestive and excretive systems.

Sounds to me like the short term plan is killing the long term plan with an axe! Always keep short term and long term plans in tact, never sacrificing one for the other. Oh, yeah, and parents: Want to have kids that don't have defects and diseases? You're not doing it right. Want to eat food that doesn't have mutated cells? You're not doing it right. The pepperoni on your nuked pizza has nitrates that will glow in the dark when you take it out of your nuker. Seriously, your frozen chicken dinner entrée that suddenly became unfrozen and over-cooked is just that—over-cooked about 1000 times.

That's how the cell-structure is altered. Get out your lead blanket if you want to live. Food corporations nuke food thousands of times more intensely than home microwaves to eliminate food impurities. But that's not all they kill. So spin that little tray table round and round in your nuker, that way you're sure to nuke all the food cells, cells that are already so full of hormones and antibiotics they're bound to mutate, change, and turn to attack.

Ever notice that your nuked food will be burning hot—actually scalding hot in one spot, yet somehow still cold in another? It's been mutated. Just some parts way more than others. Don't eat it. Just don't eat it. It's that simple. You have a choice.

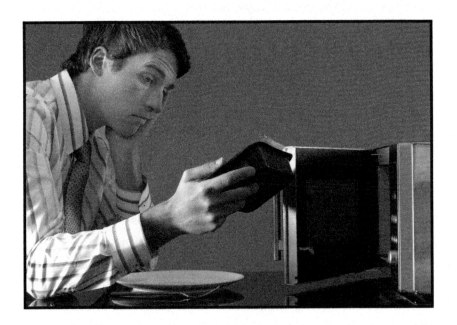

How and why microwave ovens cause cancer

Mainstream medicine fails to make the connection between microwaveable foods and cancer because Orthodox medicine thinks nutrition and diet have nothing to do with disease. This is sad but true. Most medicine today focuses on *germs and genes*, and that's it. Intervention is based on *man-made drugs or surgical procedures*, and if you want more proof, just check out most hospital food. At the hospital, there are microwave ovens (radiation ranges).

Agitated molecules

Nutritionists know that heating food kills the nutrients, including enzymes, especially once heated over 118 degrees. There are exceptions to this rule of thumb, but not many. However, even though you may be broiling, boiling, or baking, you are not necessarily creating carcinogenic food, as you are with microwaving. Normal cooking heats food from the outside in. This is the normal function of thermal dynamics. Basically, the heat transfers to cold. However, microwave radiation does just the opposite and heats from the inside out. How could this be?

All microwave ovens contain a magnetron, which is a tube in which electrons are affected by magnetic and electric fields. They produce micro wavelength radiation at about 2450 Mega Hertz (MHz) or 2.45 Giga Hertz (GHz). Microwave ovens use electromagnetic radiation to reverse the polarity of molecules, atoms and cells at *100 billion times a second*, according to research. No organic system can withstand such violent, destructive power from this kind of friction in its water molecules for any extended period of time, and not even in the "low energy range" of milliwatts. Still, this is the core function of microwave ovens - to agitate the water molecules to produce frictional heat. ***There is direct damage to cell walls and genes from microwaves.*** This is just a small glimpse of gene altering technology, and now you can imagine what the biotech industry as a whole is doing to the most popular foods and seeds, like corn, soy, alfalfa and canola. It is the technology of breaking cells, extinguishing the very life of the cells by neutralizing the electrical potentials.

Radiolytic compounds are created by microwaving organic matter. These are also created by normal cooking, but not nearly to the same extent. By using microwave ovens regularly, especially to cook meals and side dishes that take four to ten minutes to cook, you are modifying the cellular activity in your own body. Your healthy cells are forced into emergency mode by the damaged cells and the radiolytic compounds. Your cells are forced into anaerobic energy production, and *no longer have normal cellular oxidation*. This, my friends, is a cancerous condition. It's not so hard to do the math now is it? Stop using microwave ovens. Keep your cells normal and organic.

http://www.naturalnews.com/030651_microwave_cooking_cancer.html

Radiation ovens and the curse of convenience

It turns out it was the Nazis who actually invented microwave ovens. They were used in their mobile support calling them the *radiomissor*. These ovens were to be used for the invasion of Russia, because by using electronic equipment for preparation of meals on a mass scale, the logistical problem of cooking fuels would have been eliminated, as well as the convenience of producing edible products in a greatly reduced time-factor. Also, after the war, the Allies discovered medical research done by the Germans on microwave ovens.

These documents, along with some working microwave ovens, were transferred to the United States War Department and classified for reference and further scientific investigation. At the time, the Soviets issued an international warning on the health hazards, both biological and environmental, of microwave ovens and similar frequency electronic devices. Carcinogens were formed in virtually all foods tested. No test food was subjected to more microwaving than necessary to accomplish the purpose, such as cooking, thawing, or heating to ensure sanitary ingestion. This research is concrete yet it is not shared in the mainstream because *nukers* are big business in the U.S.

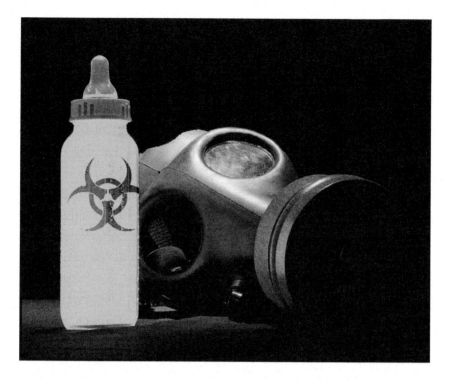

Want to know what your radiation oven is really setting you up for?

1. Microwaving milk and cereal grains converts amino acids into carcinogens.

2. Thawing frozen fruits converts glucoside and galactoside into carcinogenic substances.

3. Extremely short exposure of raw, cooked or frozen vegetables converts their plant alkaloids into carcinogens.

4. Carcinogenic free radicals are formed in microwaved plants, especially root vegetables.

One short-term study found significant and disturbing changes in the blood of individuals consuming microwaved milk and vegetables. Similar molecule agitation or isolation is used in pharmaceutical drug labs and by the biotech (GMO) food industry. The bottom line is that every microwave oven leaks electromagnetic radiation, harms food, and converts substances to dangerous organ-toxic products. It makes no sense that the FDA has not banned them altogether, along with genetically modified seeds. Microwave ovens are in ninety percent of American households. Watch out especially when you nuke organic things, like milk, meat and vegetables. The cells change, like in a bad horror movie, and then, you eat them. For that test, actual humans have volunteered as lab rats, and the facts are in. It has been diagnosed in humans that using microwave ovens extensively leads to malfunctions within the lymphatic system. Cancer causing free radicals break down your tissue and metamorphasize.

Most Cancer Linked to Diet

Seventy percent of all cancers are diet related, coming in just second to tobacco as the most influential factor in the development of cancer. Diet related. It's the chemical substances in our foods that act as mutagens or cancer promoters.

Nitrates in deli meats like salami, pastrami, turkey, and ham and the beloved, "high quality" bologna, are all converted in your body to nitrosamines, which are potent carcinogens. Never nuke hot dogs or other foods high in nitrates, because it compounds the issue of carcinogens at an exponential rate. Pesticides on your fruit and vegetables, and saccharin as your sugar substitute are also major players in your "gradual" corrosion. Especially when you microwave these foods and then eat them, the genetic code of your blood's DNA can be—and is being-- altered, and these abnormal cells are encouraged by your chemical intake to multiply, travel, and sometimes re-generate. That's metastasis. The best reversal of this is to eat the right fats and foods that are rich in omega 3's, and then alkalize the body with real spring water and organic fruits and vegetables, which will counter the previous influx you've experienced with unaltered, non-poisoned vitamins, nutrients and minerals. this alone can stop the damage - stop the bleeding.

Go for the Roots!

Free radicals—the reactive compounds that damage tissues and start cancers by promoting tumor growth have a nemesis called Beta Carotene. These antioxidants protect the body from the free radicals by helping the system build immunity, and then cancer cells are less likely to multiply and win the battle. Do it—fortify your cell membranes so they are less vulnerable to attacks.

Understanding exactly what microwave ovens due to your food and your body is crucial to not eating cancer food. Simply put, radiation is the result of nuclear decay. In basic terms, a microwave oven decays the molecular structure of the food and the packaging in which many items are cooked—by using radiation. Had the manufacturers named them radiation ovens, it's very doubtful they would be popular today.

What's the solution? Get rid of the microwave oven right now, and just deal with cleaning your own safe pot or stainless steel pan. Then drastically reduce your use of plastic. Look for natural alternatives like textiles, solid wood, bamboo, and glass.

http://www.naturalnews.com/034101_microwaveable_containers_plastics.
html#ixzz2aXcPCNQW

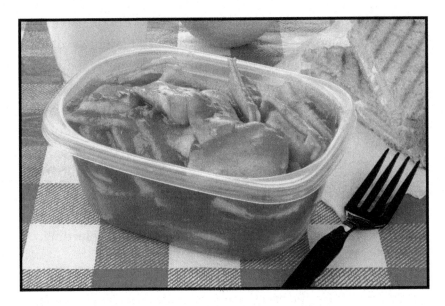

Microwave containers leach toxins into food at alarming rates

You know how they say microwave a potato in plastic wrap to hold in the moisture? What about the instructions on boxes that say cut holes in the plastic wrap? What is used to make the boxes, the containers, the plastic, the coloring chemicals, what about when that creeps into your food. New research reveals those toxins to be far greater than ever anticipated., Plastic, cellophane, cardboard and Styrofoam: Since most containers do not visibly melt or get hot, consumers have the false notion that the synthetic boxes and wrappers are not releasing toxins, but new research shows they are, and at levels that are alarming. Consumers are guaranteeing a *triple* dose of poison when they buy processed food, which contains synthetic ingredients, "nuke" them in a microwave, and then consume the *radiated chemicals and vapors* from the packaging.

The FDA claims that if some product is labeled microwave safe, then it's fine, but there are several major gray areas being exploited. The FDA also says that microwave-safe plastic wrap should never directly touch the food. The labels on many plastic wraps recommend a one inch space between the plastic and the food, but it's all locked in the oven with your food anyway.

For starters, chemical migration from packaging material to a food does not require direct contact. Excessive heat applied to the container drives off the chemical gases from the container. It is now proven that chemicals like BPA, Bisphenol-A, seep out of the container and affect humans, causing hormonal imbalances, lowered sperm count, and various other forms of cancer.

Watch out for rubber lids and their containers. Also put on the caution list freezer bags which can emit phthalates and BPA. The amount of toxins released from the synthetic depends on how long you freeze or cook them, and also the strength of each particular microwave oven. Meat trays, foam containers, coated cardboard, and most soup and noodle cups top the danger list. It is very common to cover a plate of food with plastic wrap.. These methods are not safe at all.

The FDA claims that leached substances pose no threat to a person's health. They say to use containers and materials that are specifically labeled as microwave-safe, but not to microwave margarine tubs and carryout containers from restaurants.

That brings us to research the difference between margarine tubs and all other plastic containers. Some plastics marked with recycle codes 3 or 7 can actually be made with BPA. Yogurt, butter, margarine, cottage cheese, sour cream, and many more similar foods are all sold in plastic containers, many of which are made from polypropylene (plastic # 5), one of the least-recyclable plastics. Most city recycling centers won't even accept it!

How can the FDA allow toxic chemicals in food containers that are not recyclable? Understanding this is important to realizing the true betrayal we face with the FDA. In other words, it is not acceptable to incur the expense of sorting, collecting, cleaning and reprocessing containers, but it is acceptable that we treat millions of Americans with chemotherapy after *eating* cancer. Radiation is the result of nuclear decay. In simplest terms, a microwave oven decays the molecular structure of the food and packaging by using radiation. Had the manufacturers named them *radiation ovens*, it's very doubtful they would be popular today.

Know these facts:

- Eating food processed from a microwave oven causes permanent brain damage by shorting out electrical impulses in the brain.
- Male and female hormone production is shut down and/or altered by continually eating microwaved foods.
- Minerals, vitamins, and nutrients of all microwaved food is reduced or altered so that the human body gets little or no benefit.
- The minerals in vegetables are altered into cancerous free-radicals when cooked in nukers.
- Microwaved foods cause stomach and intestinal cancerous tumors.
- Continual ingestion of microwaved food lowers the immune system.
- Eating microwaved food causes loss of memory, concentration, emotional instability, and a decrease of intelligence.

Microwaved foods lower the body's ability to utilize B-complex vitamins, Vitamin C, Vitamin E, essential minerals.

http://www.naturalnews.com/023103_microwave_food_microwaved.html#ixzz2cEV3m5gm

Modern mainstream medicine cannot fathom a connection with microwave foods to cancer. Orthodox medicine thinks nutrition and diet have nothing to do with disease because it is focused only on germs and genes. Their intervention is based on man-made drugs or surgical procedures. Check out hospital food as a partial confirmation of this philosophy. Hospitals serve up processed foods, artificial sweeteners, foods loaded with hydrogenated, processed GMO oils like corn, canola and cottonseed, and they even serve these foods to patients who are dying.

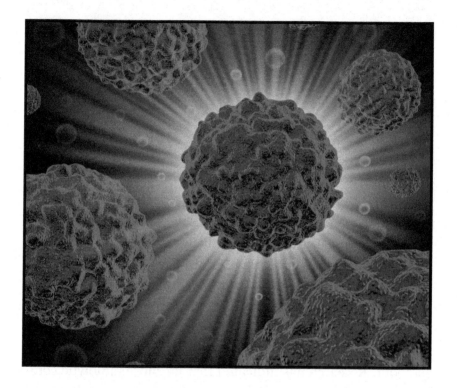

Agitated Molecules and Warped Cells

Baking, broiling or frying food heats it from the outside in. This is the normal function of thermal dynamics: heat transfers to cold. Although cooking most food at heat higher than 118 degrees kills most of the nutrients, especially enzymes, microwave cooking does much more damage because the radiation heats the food from the inside out. Now of course, you want to know how it does that. Let's examine.

Electromagnetic radiation creates an alternating current, which reverses the polarity of the atoms, molecules and cells up to one hundred billion times per second. This destructive power is violent in that the water molecules and their structures are literally torn apart and forcefully deformed, which is called struc-

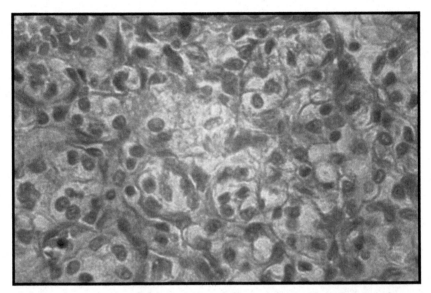

tural isomerism. The agitation of the water molecules produces frictional heat, and this is why certain parts of the food will be piping hot, but others remain cold. The friction is unpredictable, and so are microwave ovens.

There is direct damage occurring to cell walls and genes from microwaves. Gene altering technology is exactly what GMO is all about. Research has indicated that far more radiolytic compounds are created by microwave cooking. This weakens the human immune system, neutralizing the electrical potentials of the very life of our cells, leading to the development of mutated cells. In other words, the human cells are forced from normal cellular oxidation into the anaerobic energy production of glucose fermentation. *This is a cancerous condition.* Cancer cells thrive when normal cells are deprived of oxygen. This is why cancer patients should not eat refined sugar, artificial sweeteners, or genetically modified hydrogenated oils.

http://www.naturalnews.com/030651_microwave_cooking_cancer. html#ixzz2cEkoiy41

The Solution

What's the solution? Nuke the nuker! Axe it. 86 it! Get rid of it. Get rid of the microwave oven right now, and just deal with cleaning your own safe pot or stainless steel pan. Then drastically reduce your use of plastic. Look for natural alternatives like textiles, solid wood, bamboo, and glass. Change your daily intake. Change what you cook and what you use to cook on and in. It's time to stop eating cancer.

http://environment.about.com/od/reducingwaste/a/corn_plastic.htm

http://www.riversideonline.com/health_reference/Cancer/AN00873.cfm

http://healthychild.org/5steps/5_steps_5/?gclid=CLuk4pDLnawCFQsj7AodV...

http://curezone.com/foods/microwave_oven_risk.asp

http://www.naturalnews.com/034101_microwaveable_containers_plastics.html#ixzz2c2bChyYT

http://www.naturalnews.com/034101_microwaveable_containers_plastics.html#ixzz2c2awTQcm

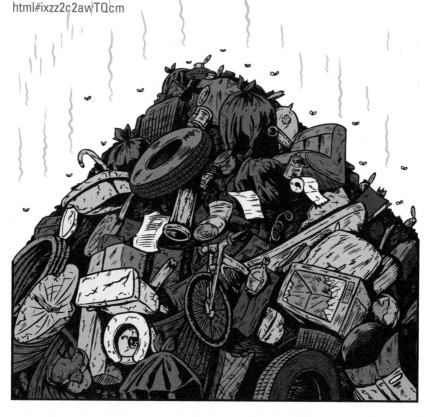

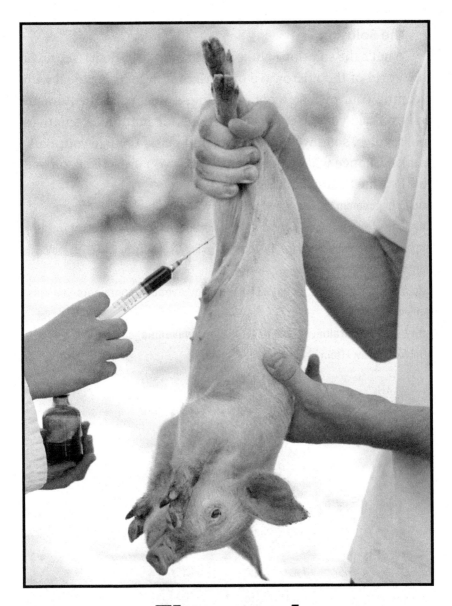

Chapter 4
Hormone Injections in Animals

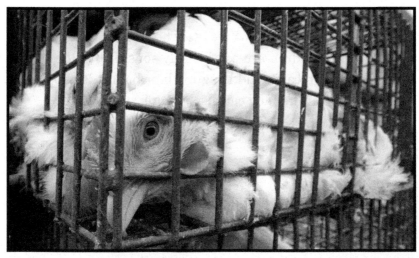

Hormones make pigs, chickens, and cows fatter and meatier, but they are the driving force for breast cancer and prostate cancer. Hormones breed tumors that kill its consumers. Smart consumers eat only farm-raised animals that are free of antibiotics and hormones because they know the difference. Beware! Eating chemicals is more popular now than ever before, and the corporations using them to beef up your food are richer than ever in our history. Please, you deserve to live to appreciate everything you've done in this life that's gotten you this far! Be the greatest guard at the temple of your very own soul. Keep the poisonous intruders from ever entering. It's your duty and your obligation.

Hormones in Meat Linked to Cancer Risk

Artificial hormones in U.S. beef have been linked to breast cancer and prostate cancer. There is new concern over evidence that growth and sex hormones in beef can cause genital abnormalities in boys, and early onset of puberty in girls. Approximately two thirds of all cattle in the U.S. are pumped full of hormones. Hormones like progesterone, testosterone, oestradiol and zeranol are known to disrupt the body's natural balance, causing all sorts of biological effects. Oestradiol is considered to be a cancer risk.

Breast cancer is much more prominent for U.S. women than it is for European women, where these hormones are banned for use in cattle. Children are particularly sensitive to these hormones which can cause sudden growth or breast development. Remember, boys and men can also get breast cancer.

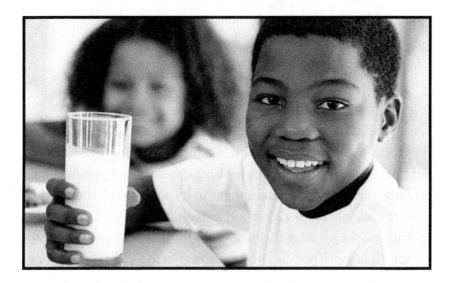

Hormones in Milk Linked to Cancer Risk

Did you hear the latest? Even WalMart bans rBGH tainted milk! Why? WalMart is the latest in a string of large retailers to recognize the consumer demand for milk from cows not treated with recombinant bovine growth hormone (rBGH). The Walmart store brand milk, Great Value, will now come from dairies that have pledged not to use rBGH. Sam's Club will also begin offering milk choices from cows not treated with the hormone. Major retailers like Kroger and Safeway are also changing their store brands over. Even Starbucks has followed suit with non-rBGH milk. Now that says something!

However, despite this good news from some of the major retailers, most conventional, non-organic milk in this country still comes from cows treated with rBGH, a genetically engineered hormone designed to increase a cow's milk production and earn larger profits for dairies, all at the risk of human health. The FDA approved the use of rBGH in 1993, but since then, several substantial independent scientific studies conclude it does pose a serious risk to human health. Other studies contradict these findings; however they tend to be produced by the industries that benefit from the use of rBGH. Go figure! That's like leaving the fox in charge of the hen house.

How do hormones in animals affect humans that consume the by-products?

Independent scientists have studied the effects of rBGH on health and the use of this hormone is a serious potential risk factor for cancer. Milk from cows treated with rBGH contains significantly higher levels of a hormone: insulin-like growth factor-1 (IGF-1). Experiments have shown that at higher than normal biological levels, IGF-1 is linked to cancer in humans, particularly cancers of the breast and prostate, but also others. Why is that? IGF-1 is similar in structure to insulin. It stimulates cell division and plays an important role in childhood growth. So where's the problem? IGF-1 in milk from rBGH treated cows may have up to twenty times the normal levels of IGF-1. Furthermore, there is evidence that the IGF-1 found in milk as a result of rBGH use is a more truncated form which may be up to 40 times more potent than naturally occurring IGF-1, and it can wreak havoc on our cellular signaling systems.

Infants and children may be even more susceptible to the harmful effects of high levels of IGF-1 because of their smaller blood plasma volume. Some scientists have even suggested that future cancers could be "seeded" in youngsters exposed to high levels of IGF-1 in hormone treated milk.

Twenty years of research show the dangers of hormone-laden milk

More than twenty years of research have proven that IGF-1 can initiate or promote cancer in the cell. In 1992, the New England Journal of Medicine acknowledged that the class of hormones to which IGF-1 belongs is one of the factors responsible for normal breast tissue developing into cancerous tissue. Higher than normal blood levels of IGF-1 are related to an increased risk of breast, prostate, and colon cancers. Accumulating scientific evidence has been enough for other governments of the world to prohibit the use of rBGH, including Canada, the European Union and Japan. Unfortunately, the FDA has not followed suit.

The myths get busted about IGF-1

Food-drug pushers will often claim the following: "IGF-1 is naturally occurring." Well, yes, that's true, IGF-1 is naturally occurring, but so is poison ivy, but we don't use that in food. They also claim that "IGF-1 in milk cannot be absorbed by the human gut." This is simply not true. In both humans and rats, studies have shown that many proteins, including IGF-1, are absorbed intact into the blood stream. Infants are even more susceptible! rBGH makes cows suffer from over stretched udders which can easily become infected. This in turn leads to higher levels of antibiotics used by the farmers. Do you see the vicious cycle now? No wonder there are "superbugs" in hospitals now that antibiotics can't beat back. Humans are quickly becoming immune to all classes of antibiotics, thanks to this style of CAFO, abusive farming.

Many small farms and organic farmers do not use hormones at all. Always ask questions and read the labels. Natural News.com is a great resource for knowing which companies still have morals and ethics and the ones that do not put money and profits before consumer health.

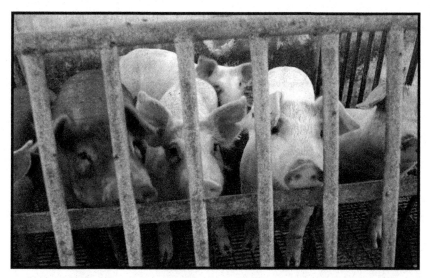

Majority of U.S. pork tainted with deadly drugs, bacteria

The next time you reach for the bacon, ham, pork chops or pork steaks, you may want to rethink your dining choice: A majority of samples of the other white meat that were obtained in a recent study contained bacteria, potentially deadly drugs or a combination of both. According to Consumer Reports, samples of U.S. pork chops and ground pork were found to contain substantial amounts of harmful, antibiotic-resistant bacteria, along with low levels of a type of growth hormone used on pigs. A bacterium that can cause fever, diarrhea, and abdominal pain, was widespread. Some samples harbored other potentially harmful bacteria, including salmonella. Why is this so alarming? Some of the bacteria found by the CR investigation were resistant to antibiotics that are commonly used to treat humans. These are grave implications in the scope of overall healthcare.

The True Nightmare of CAFOs: Confined Animal Feeding Operations

Dirty conditions can allow bacteria to proliferate, which is often the case when large-scale production facilities confine animals in close quarters – hence the expression/acronym – CAFO.

Recent lab research done by Boston University indicated that repeated low doses of antibiotics can cause enough stress in bac-

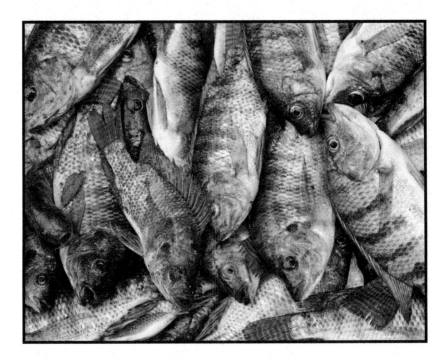

teria to increase the rate of spontaneous mutations, eventually rendering the (super) bugs drug-resistant - a process known as mutagenesis.

Farm raised fish sounds good, but usually means the same as CAFO

Farm raised with regards to fish, like tilapia, often means ponds that are overcrowded, laden with ammonia and bacteria, and then pumped full of growth hormones and other GMO for desired production results that quantify higher profits. For example, tampering with the genes of a popular fish to make it twice as large is sick and demented. Plus, GM salmon can breed with other fish and pass on the messed up genes. (http://www. organicconsumers.org/articles/article_27667.cfm)

Did you hear about GM tilapia too? Here's some recent

research: "Tilapia fish engineered for transgenic expression of growth hormone had deformed heads and backs, atrophied gonads, and lower mineral content"

http://natureinstitute.org/nontarget/reports/tilapia_001.php

People are already frustrated and overwhelmed with food choices, and some people still think farm raised fish means some "pond" farmer took good care of them, but it's just the opposite, they are feeding them hormones and pumping the lake full of antibiotics to kill the disease that spreads from population and fish feces overload. This is like breeding cancer and auto-immune disorder on purpose! Maybe tadpoles and squid won't be enough feed for this new mutated fish species. Picture these Franken-salmon in huge tanks, existing in some biotech, heavily guarded warehouses in America, just waiting to be released into our great oceans, so they can tear into some other salmon, and eat other fish salmon would never eat, and kill animals salmon would not kill, like all the humans who consume them now.

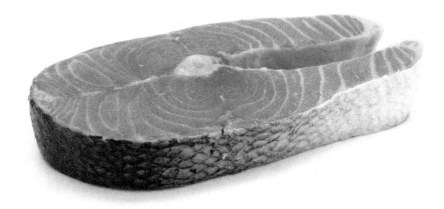

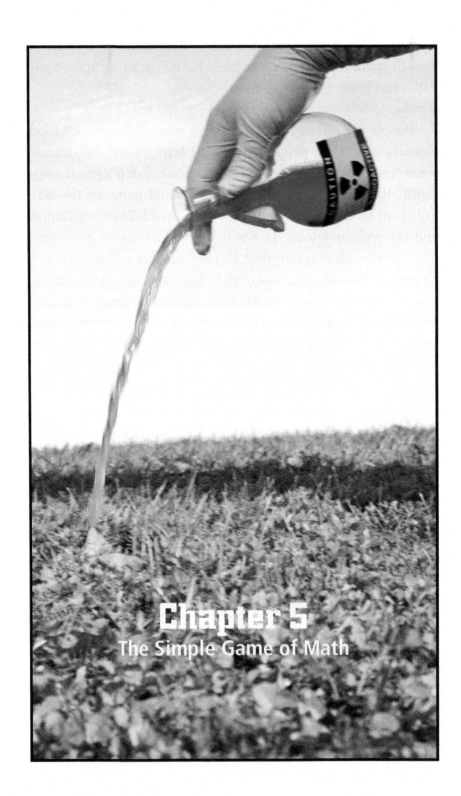

Chapter 5
The Simple Game of Math

Today, we are reviewing simple arithmetic. Get your thinking caps on for this one. Here we go. In math, if you add 2 + 2 + 2 + 2 + 2 + 2 + 2 + 2, you get 16.

Trivia: Can you add up the following eight words to get a simple answer? Their definitions come from the dictionary.

Food: material taken into an organism and used for nourishment, growth, repair, and vital processes; a source of energy.
Agent: a means; an instrument; proxy.
Synthetic: not genuine; produced artificially, esp. by chemical means.
Chemical: a substance used for producing a chemical effect.
By-Product: something produced in addition to the main product.
Carcinogen: an agent causing or inciting cancer.
Mutation: a sudden or relatively permanent change in a hereditary character.
Corrosion: to eat or be eaten away gradually, as by action of rust or of a chemical.
(answer on the next page)

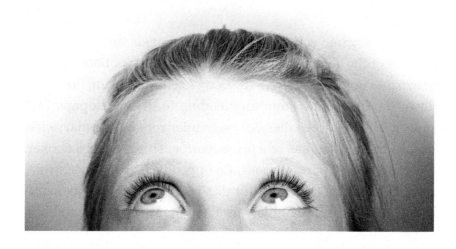

Answer: That's right kids ... the grand total equals

Cancer!

And now you have the keys to its prevention.

Now, what else do we know about this silent serial killer? Cancer (noun) has a few simple definitions: One is *A harmful growth in the body caused when cells increase without control; often known as an evil that spreads and brings destruction.* Then there is this definition: *A cancer on society, or a cancerous war; or to cancel with cancer; to cancel life early.* You see, cancer cancels life, after you've worked and slaved half a lifetime to make yourself somebody, in hopes that one day you wouldn't have to work, and the world would be at your side, waiting for you to enjoy it to the fullest. Isn't there something we should have been watching out for all this time, something that weakens us a little bit each day that goes by, setting us up for a fall. The perception is that there's no cure, and for many already sick with the disease that is true. But for many others the illness can be avoided by following some common-sense advice.

Beware of Additives and "Preservatives"
You read on labels everywhere that call sodium benzoate *a preservative.* But those warning labels should say "a preservative that kills."

Savvy organic consumers and nutritionists may know, but the rest of the general population does not know about sodium benzoate's ability to deprive the body's cells of oxygen, breaking down the immune system and leading to the development of cancer. This stealthy killer is flying under consumer radar, with its user friendly tagline, as a *preservative.* This silent cell choker has found its way into thousands of products, even foods that are labeled as *all natural.* But don't be fooled. While benzoic acid is found naturally in low levels in many fruits, the sodium benzoate listed on a product's label is synthesized in a lab.

Derived from a reaction of benzoic acid with sodium hydroxide, sodium benzoate is actually the sodium salt of benzoic acid. Sodium benzoate is a known carcinogenic additive which, when eaten or applied to the skin, gets transported to the liver, where it is supposed to be filtered, and eventually expelled in urine, but the damage gets done before that process is completed.

Sodium benzoate chokes out your body's nutrients at the DNA/cellular level by depriving mitochondria of oxygen, sometimes completely shutting them down. Just as humans need oxygen to breathe, cells need oxygen to function   properly and to fight off infection, including cancer. The FDA says it's safe because the amount used to preserve foods is very low, but don't ever combine it with vitamin C or E, or benzene is formed. Danger! Benzene is a known carcinogen, which means it causes cancer. So now why is it put in food? It's the cheapest mold inhibiter on the market, so it's all about the money. Acidic foods tend to grow bacteria, mold and yeast more easily than non-acidic foods, so the sodium benzoate extends the shelf life, while it shortens human life.

Cancer is all about the cumulative effect. When the human body is exposed repeatedly to any level of this carcinogen, which now rears its ugly head in thousands of products, the immune system, over time, is depleted to the point that one acquires an immune deficiency. Then the body does not have enough essential nutrients to detoxify, and this occurs at the cellular level. Parkinson's, neuro-degenerative diseases, and premature aging have all been attributed to this infamous preservative. Also, watch out for BHA, BHT and EDTA.

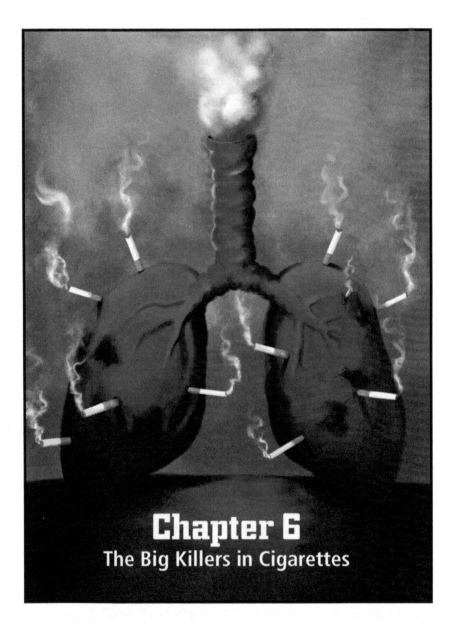

Chapter 6
The Big Killers in Cigarettes

And The Best Killer Ingredient Awards Go To:

Gold Medal: <u>Ammonia</u>: keeps the smokers addicted to more than just the "NIC FIT" of it. It actually makes the nicotine exponentially potent.

Silver Medal: <u>Pesticide/Herbicide</u>: keeps the bugs and weeds off of corporate tobacco; means more to sell.

Bronze Medal: <u>Fiberglass</u>, yes, like in your attic. It burns hotter so your cigarette doesn't go out when the wind blows.

Honorable Mention: <u>Tar</u>, which helps the cancer lodge in your lungs.

These big four have killed more than a half million people in 2013.

When you compare corporate killings to the horror of the thousands that have died in Iraq and Afghanistan —it's like corporate cancer is a form of genocide. It's erasing the people who don't make a daily effort to filter out these corporate-fueled "easy-money chemicals" from their food because they just don't know better. And it's all done by corporations to widen profit margins. So when they say, "it's not about the money," you know it always is. You can escape the jail of cancer by boycotting the chemicals sold as foods today. There's a new chemical war going on, and the educated consumers are fighting back.

Win the War of Attrition

Epithelial tissue is what lines the inside and outside of our bodies. It's thin and very susceptible to damage. Think of the skin in your mouth, your throat, the lining in your lungs, your stomach, your colon, and your prostate, if you still have one. Imagine what cigarettes and cigars do to the lining of your lungs. Carbon monoxide, nitrogen oxides, hydrogen cyanide and ammonia are all present in cigarette smoke. These thin layers of skin and lining are very exposed to what can abrade them and wear them down by irritation, burning, or constant brushing with chemicals and their agents. Our skin is our largest organ, and it absorbs chemicals easily—they go right into our bloodstream. As a habitual smoker, it's going to be very tough for your lungs to fight off gangs of mutant cells.

Pouring insecticide and weed killer on your lawn allows your pets to step in it, then the skin on their paws actually absorbs it; and they can contract leukemia when they're less than six years old. It happened to my cat. Don't eat cancer, or smoke it, and don't put it on you or your pet's skin either. You and your dog deserve a long life.

Ammonia in Cigarettes—Oh, you didn't know?!

Ammonia is added in the form of ammonium hydroxide or diammonium phosphate. There is no regulation on this. Yes, we know cigarettes are bad for you, but why are the manufacturers allowed to cook in ammonia? Big Tobacco is the answer to that question. Big Tobacco has been running that show since the late 1960's and early 1970's. Remember R.J. Reynolds? Remember when *Marlboro* and *Kool* nearly put all the others out of business? Here is why ammonia has been used in smoking products:

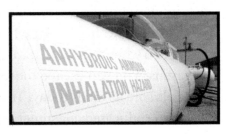

Added to present nicotine in a free-based form in the smoke.

Speeds up and increases nicotine's hit.

Reduces amount of nicotine measured by the smoking machine tests.

The nicotine hits your brain faster.

The addiction is stronger and harder to beat.

Nicotine levels on cigarette packs don't actually tell you the amount of nicotine you'll get if you smoke that cigarette. Big Tobacco lobbyists like that one. Attention chain smokers: *You're addicted to free-based nicotine!* Ammonia turns normal nicotine into free-based nicotine. This process is similar to one used to heighten the effects of cocaine, in a drug you may have heard of called crack, and can boost the availability of nicotine up to one hundred times. Free-based nicotine is already in a gas form, so once it's in the lungs, it moves quickly into the bloodstream and to waiting nicotine receptors. Without ammonia, nicotine in burned tobacco smoke is a solid, tiny particle that must travel on the smoke stream into the smoker's lungs, and there is absorbed more slowly. Ammonia in the cigarette increases the pH of the smoke and turns some of the nicotine solid into a gas. This means that with ammonia included, the same amount of nicotine will have a stronger physiological effect on the smoker.

Marlboro and *Kool* brands saw a dramatic increase in their market share when they began to include ammonia. Now ammonia is a common ingredient, usually found in the form of ammonium hydroxide. Look for it in your next pack on the box. Free-based nicotine (the crack of all nicotine) is not detectable on the standard smoking machine that the U.S. government has used for measuring the tar and nicotine content of cigarette brands.

Adding ammonia to a cigarette brand causes its measured nicotine levels to go down, while in fact delivering at least the same amount of nicotine and in a more highly-addictive method. Smokers who try to wean themselves from their nicotine addiction by selecting low-nicotine brands are not getting accurate numbers, and may actually be choosing a more addictive product.

Tobacco companies began adding ammonia compounds to cigarettes in the 1960s to boost the effect of nicotine on hooking smokers, according to an expert witness in Minnesota's lawsuit against the tobacco industry. The state said that in 1965, scientists at R.J. Reynolds were trying to find out why their Winston brand was losing ground to Philip Morris' Marlboro brand, and in their research discovered that Marlboro contained ammonia compounds. In the 1970s, Reynolds started adding ammonia and slowly but surely, everyone fell in line. By 1990, documents showed that tobacco companies were using more than ten million pounds of ammonia compounds each year.

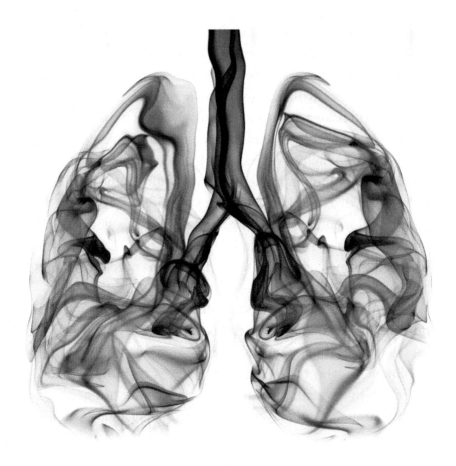

Chapter 7
Secret Lethal Ingredient

If a cigarette filter was simply made of cotton and paper, and you threw it out in the yard, it would break up and disintegrate after a couple of rainstorms. Of course, that doesn't happen. Why?

Fiberglass became popular in the United States in the early 1990's as asbestos was phased out. Asbestos is like fiberglass in that it doesn't evaporate in the air, dissolve in water or react with most chemicals. Tiny glass particles are wrapped and bound tightly in filters to keep some of the tar from entering

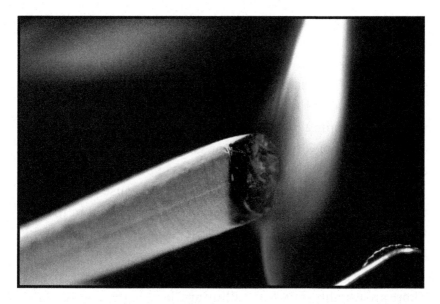

your mouth, but many of these microscopic fibers escape into your mouth, throat and lungs.

The x-ray of lung cancer patients looks like ground glass is sitting at the bottom of each lung. Think now of why filters take up to fifteen years to disintegrate. It all adds up. Also, fiberglass has the heat-resistant qualities that made asbestos so desirable for insulation. It acts as a buffer to heat. Now you know why *your fingertips never even get warm, much less hot, when you smoke a cigarette* all the way down to the filter. Consider this: If you have ever been in an attic and got insulation on your skin, you already know those tiny fibers of glass from insulation wool can irritate your skin very badly, and also cause problems with your eyes. If you experience too much contact with fiberglass, it can cause what's called irritant contact dermatitis, or inflammation of the skin. This happens inside the lungs of smokers, increasing the difficulty of breathing. Fiberglass is nothing more than glass wool rolled into bunches for insulating homes. Fiberglass can be just as dangerous as asbestos—and is sometimes referred to as the asbestos of the 21st century. A study in 1970 on rats stated that fibrous glass of small diameter is a potent carcinogen, leading to changes in the DNA genetic structure and breaking down the immune system.

Just think about the inside of your cheeks and the softness of the tissue. That same soft tissue coats your throat and lungs. The carbon rod at the tip of the cigarette is insulated and bound with two wrapping mats of glass fibers. Discharged glass fibers and glass particles from the filter go into the smoker's mouth, and subsequently, the bio-resistant glass fibers and microscopic glass dust are inhaled and ingested. This can cause tiny rips and tears in the lung's lining, which is like spilling blood in the water for the sharks to feed upon. Escape the prison of poisonous smoke, and your body will celebrate the change.

The success rates for smokers trying to quit are dismal. There are roughly forty five million smokers in the United States alone, and half of them want to quit. Only five percent will succeed without some form of help. Most return to smoking within six months. That is a cold hard fact. The scary commercials only help about four percent quit, reports the CDC. The pills and the patch only help about ten percent to quit, if they're lucky, and electronic cigarettes, better known as e-cigs help even fewer smokers kick the habit altogether because most people remain addicted to nicotine, which is still highly toxic to cleansing organs like the liver and pancreas.

One of the main reasons quitting rates are so dismal is that the juiced up nicotine in commercial grade cigarettes enters the bloodstream easier as it rides in as a vapor, where your epithelial (soft) tissues are being destroyed, over and over again, by tiny shards of glass wool, mixed with the tar—this is all just sealed into place. The secret lethal ingredient is an evil scheme, to keep smokers literally stuck in a vicious cycle of temporarily relieving anxiety and depression with nicotine. I call it the cigarette hangover, which is just one part of the *14 And Out* program that I designed in order to help smokers understand this, so they know what they are quitting, not just how and why.

The lesson teaches you exactly what to do during the first fourteen days, step by step. I am very direct and practical here with the strategies, because this is where most smokers fall off when they try to quit, during the first two weeks. That is why the program is called *14 And Out*, because you are basically weaned off nicotine and the total habit of smoking in fourteen days, or sometimes less. Some people quit cold turkey immediately after they finish the sixty minute lesson or read the book. Because the class involves hands on activities which shock the student about what's really inside a cigarette, I invite you to dissect one cigarette while reading *14 And Out* and follow along as I take you on a quick journey through all the major chemicals you find in one typical commercial cigarette, including bleach, ammonia, glass wool and plastic.

When you combine this vicious cocktail of toxins and burn them, you are creating your own vicious cycle which uses nicotine as the aspirin relief from the chemical hangover. *14 And Out* could be your way out of this vicious cycle.

Here's the link to the free preview/trailer of *14 And Out* presented by the Health Ranger Mike Adams:

http://premium.naturalnews.tv/14AndOut__TV.htm

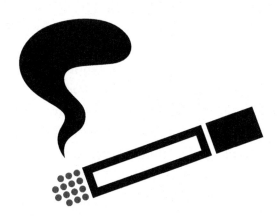

Chapter 8
Breathing in Fiberglass and Plastic

Glass wool, fiberglass, fibrous glass, and glass fibers are all names for the same thing: thin, needle-shaped rods of glass, which nature does not make, but humans do. Fiberglass is now causing serious health concerns among U.S. officials and health researchers. Glass fibers less than 3 micrometers in diameter and greater than 20 micrometers in length are potent carcinogens in rats. Studies have continued to show that fibers of this size not only cause cancer in laboratory animals, but also cause changes in the activity and chemical composition of cells, leading to changes in the genetic structure and in the cellular immune system. How can this not apply to mankind? It does.

We all know, and it has been proven in humans, that breathing in asbestos is deadly and fuels cancer. In just that same light, cancer of the pleura (the outer casing of the lungs in humans) is called mesothelioma and it is caused by asbestos fibers. When glass fibers are manufactured as small as asbestos fibers and ingested, they cause cancer in laboratory animals just as asbestos does. Remember, asbestos is a potent human carcinogen, which will have killed an estimated half million American workers by 2020.

Also, why do cigarettes burn so hot (up to 1700 degrees), so evenly, and never go out in heavy wind? What's the trick? Cellulose acetate is a synthetic plastic substance commonly used for photo film. It burns very hot and efficiently. If cigarettes were rolled in simple paper, they would blow out in heavy winds. A smoker can drive down the highway at 55mph, hanging the cigarette out the window, and it will not go out. Also, a cigarette that is burning will not trail or canoe up one side. Once the ashes become uneven, they fall off, and even themselves out. Think about it. This is because cigarette manufacturers carefully weave plastic particles into the matting of the stem to keep it burning evenly. This explains why cigarettes burn so hot, up to 1700 degrees Fahrenheit during the drag. The cigarette companies wouldn't want your nicotine delivery device to go out a couple times before you get to the filter, or you might decide it's a waste of money and quit!

The paper stem is insulated and bound with wrapping mats of acetate, which is interwoven with paper, keeping the cigarette from burning too quickly. Rip one apart and look at it through a magnifying lens and you can see for yourself. A cigarette is a highly engineered, efficient nicotine delivery device. But you can outsmart the enemy. Shocking new research reveals that a specific type of lung cancer many smokers develop comes from tiny tears in their lung tissue caused by microscopic glass fibers, also known as glass wool, found in many conventional cigarette filters. These rips in 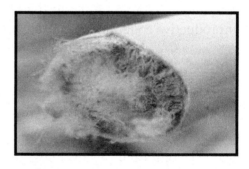 the epithelial (soft) tissue fuel the development of tumors and cancerous cells due to the constant overload of toxins, namely pesticides, nicotine and ammonia, contained in commercial cigarette smoke.

The filters of typical commercial cigarettes contain microscopic, needle-shaped shards of glass wool (like fiberglass insulation) which escape into the mouth and throat, and then lodge with tobacco tar in the lung tissue, surrounding the alveoli (tiny air sacs) and lead to COPD (chronic obstructive pulmonary disease), emphysema and eventually lung cancer.

Several medical professionals, including a radiologist at a major hospital, reviewed the damaged lung tissue of several cigarette smokers and said the x-rays looked identical to those of patients exposed to asbestos, and that diagnostic imaging revealed what looked like ground glass which settled in the soft tissue near the bottom of the lungs (GGO—ground glass opacity). The interviewed nurse said, "When lung tissue is damaged over and over, it develops lesions, and the cancer plants itself in there like seeds."

http://www.appliedradiology.com

According to the doctor, the tiny shards penetrate the "lipid bi-layer, then embed in the lung tissue, causing the tissue to harden and eventually lose its ability to absorb oxygen." This damage fuels the development of the same type of lung cancer (mesothelioma) associated with asbestos poisoning. He also explained how smoking destroys the cilia (tiny hairs) that help push excretions/mucus out, and how when smokers sleep, their breathing patterns relax and the "tar deposits creep in on damaged air sacs called blebs, eventually rupturing and collapsing them." This is why when smokers awake in the morning they can experience unproductive coughing fits and/or bronchial spasms.

http://www.ncbi.nlm.nih.gov/pmc/articles/PMC1766058

Microscopic glass fibers bound in a filter

The cigarette filter (butt) acts as a buffer from the extreme heat of the cigarette's burning chemicals. Fibrous glass has the heat-resistant qualities of asbestos, which makes it an efficient material for insulation; however, if you've ever been in an attic and got insulation on your skin, you already know how irritating the glass fibers can be, so now imagine what it's doing to the inside of a smoker's lungs.

Up to twelve thousand microscopic glass fibers are tightly bound together, which explains why filters take between ten and fifteen years to disintegrate. If the filter were simply cotton rolled tightly in paper, a few rainstorms would break it up and wash it away within weeks. Filters are also constructed to catch the tar and the tobacco particles from coming through, but not entirely.

Although fiberglass is not the same as asbestos, it can be just as damaging to the human body. The long, very narrow fibers penetrate deep into lung tissue and remain there. One study conducted with rats showed that fibrous glass is a potent carcinogen, leading to changes in the DNA genetic structure and breaking down the immune system. This is one reason smoker's fight colds, the flu, sinus and bronchial infections for much longer periods of time than non-smokers.

http://tpx.sagepub.com/content/19/4-1/482.full.pdf

Independent studies reveal that commercial cigarettes with defective filters have been marketed for over sixty years. Mesothelioma, a deadly cancer that develops in the protective lining of the lungs, abdomen, and/or the cavity around the heart, is most commonly associated with asbestos poisoning, but now research reveals that more than ten of those cases are now associated with cigarette smokers with NO history of exposure to asbestos.

The tobacco industry has been negligent in failing to perform toxicological examinations to assess human health risks from inhaling and ingesting these synthetic micro-particles released from conventional cigarette filters. The recent "warning ads" about the effects of smoking are not educational, nor do they help smokers understand strategies for cessation at all. The fifty-four million dollar campaign full of stark and graphic advertisements is nothing more than a ploy to pretend like the CDC is trying to help with this massive, preventable health crisis.

http://www.cnn.com

Thanks to lax regulations regarding the ingredients used for manufacturing cigarettes, smokers are susceptible to multiple forms of lung disease, including desquamative interstitial pneumonitis from ground glass infiltration of the soft tissues, bronchoalveolar cell carcinoma, and pulmonary fibrosis, which are all revealed from specific lung biopsies (HR-CT scans).

http://www.naturalnews.com/035766_cigarettes_glass_fibers_lung_damage. html#ixzz2jiTpMBks

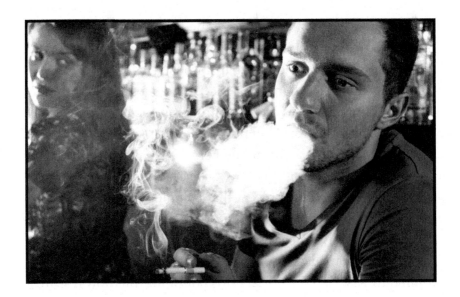

Chapter 9
The Smoker's Convention

Ever notice when you go to parties that the best conversation is always in the kitchen? It is, because that's where you'll find the drinkers. Yep. Then, after you hang out there awhile, and you mix with those wilder animals, you'll notice about a third of them will leave and head out the back, or the side door, and that's exactly when the conversation in the kitchen will lose its steam. So then, whichever you choose, to go or not to go out back with those that just left the kitchen, they won't mind, because their conversation is going to be edgy, with or without you. They are on a nicotine high, but not for long. Do you know why? They're the smokers, and they just seem to have riskier things to talk about. Plus, they're getting away from the big crowd, so they can talk about who's who, who likes who, or who's cheating on who—or who's going to cheat on who, and you wouldn't want to miss that! So get off your cell phone, and go out there, and learn something. But don't light up. On top of it all, I've noticed that the smokers, while they are smoking , seem to be generally more excited, kind of living on the edge. But when they finish that cig, you can see the look on their faces, and it tells the whole story. If you look at a smoker while they're rubbing it out, or flicking it in the yard, it seems as though they're not happy with themselves, deep down knowing that smoking a pack a day plus will probably take them out early in life.

But for some, they just feel invincible, like when we were in the middle grades, fourth to sixth, and we would take all kinds of chances, not really paying attention to consequences, because they rarely applied to us anyhow, or so we thought. And now, I bring you to the *Chemical Love Affair*. Now, thanks to the good ole' U.S. of A., most smokers are just plain addicted. For many, it started off just being a cool, relaxing thing, and now they can't walk away from the hook of the ammonia and the nicotine, or nic-fits. Sometimes, they'll hold the thing in their hands for long stretches of time, just building up that chemical love affair. They hit the pack of cigarettes on their hand about one hundred times over, or they tap that one cigarette's end to tighten up the tar and tobacco. So which is it for you? *Camel lights in a box? Menthols?! Newports? Marlboro 100's?* Most smokers don't realize that what is really relaxing them is simply a different breathing pattern than when they are not smoking.

The Zen of Breathing

Smoking gives the smoker a steady breathing pattern when they are stressed, which is part of the addiction and they don't even realize it. Too bad their air coming in is contaminated with smoke, ammonia, pesticide, and fiber glass. Heck, they'd be better off smoking weed. At least it wouldn't be tainted with chemicals. I mean, if you simply have to smoke, go buy some organic tobacco and some non-bleached cigarette paper, and roll your own.

And I've noticed, over the years, that people who do smoke usually seem more stressed than the non-smokers, just in general.

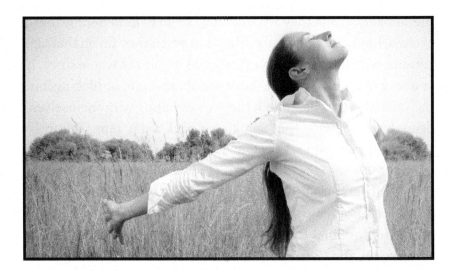

There is reason enough to quit right there. That's why their conversation is edgy, they like to get right to the point, and talk about what's bothering them, or just get to laughing so they can laugh away their issues. But then they don't even get to laugh hard, because as soon as they get to something really funny, it makes them cough that dry, raspy hack at the height of their laugh, sometimes even ruining the joke or the moment.

Are they thinking about anything when that happens? Are they thinking they might go out like that, coughing their way into a heart attack, or a stroke, or ripping apart the lining of their windpipe, to the point that all the mutagens (cancer cells) cling to the damage and finish the job for them? This sounds very harsh but it is a reality.

When I was six years old, my Grandpa Sol had smoked himself into lung cancer. My Mom said it was hard to even look at him when he got really thin, and still, he kept smoking. The doctor actually told him if he kept smoking, he would die. Was he not happy with his life? Or did he just not believe it was happening? Or maybe, just maybe, the nicotine and ammonia really weigh in more than your family, especially after years and years of cigarettes being a steady part of your days and nights? It's hard to tell. You can't ask him now.

Well, I don't know. I'm not trying to make people feel bad. I'm trying to make people feel good, about themselves, and about being aware of the chemicals that get inside them, out of habit, out of negligence, out of greed—and invade the temple, the temple of their souls. I've got my guard up all the time now. So let's dig right in. What are chemical mutagens?

Mutagens are substances that cause hereditary genetic changes or "mutations." Most mutations are harmful, and most mutagens are carcinogens. A mutagen is a natural or human-made agent (physical or chemical) which can alter the structure or sequence of DNA. This is a cold hard fact: Cancer is driven by chemical consumption. Cancer is a chemically driven killer.

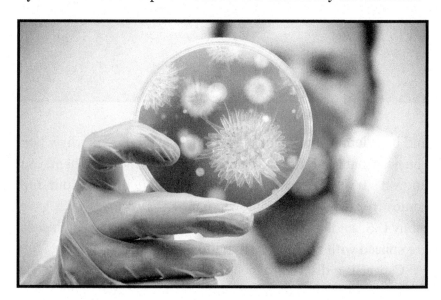

Cell mutation research dates back to World War II

The first report of mutagenic action of a chemical was in 1942 by Charlotte Auerbach, who showed that nitrogen mustard, a component of poisonous mustard gas that was used in World War I, and then in World War II by the Nazis, could cause mutations in cells. Since that time, many other mutagenic chemicals have been identified. One of the worst ever was Agent Orange used in Vietnam. Trust me, Big Food knows what causes cancer and what does not, and they've known since WWII.

Unfortunately, now, in this modern age of capitalism, we find mutagens in many food additives and skin products, and without proper regulation. All standards put on additives are based on a one hundred and seventy five pound male adult. No study I can find has ever been done in regards to how a ten or twenty pound infant would react to the same dosage.

The compounds and poisons used for pesticides are lethal

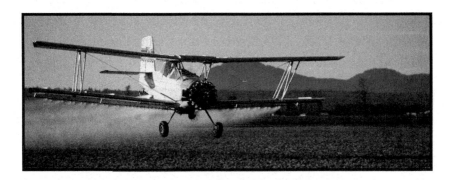

and have lethal consequences in your system, that is why when you hear that cigarettes have hundreds of chemicals in them, you know it's true. Ever heard of *Roundup Ready Crops*? Roundup comes from dioxin, also known as *Agent Orange*, which gave many U.S. soldiers cancer in Vietnam. Now tobacco plant seeds are spliced with this poison to build tolerance of it.

Cancer is a disorder of cells in the body. Your mutated cells divide, multiply, and then turn and attack your own body. It begins with a group of cells that fail to respond to the normal control mechanism and continue to divide without need. The new growths are called tumors or neoplasia and may be benign or malignant. A benign tumor is not cancerous or is one that remains localized, whereas a malignant tumor can invade neighboring tissues by entering blood vessels, especially lymphatic vessels where they can be carried to other areas of the body to form new tumors called secondaries or metastases, if not caught in time.

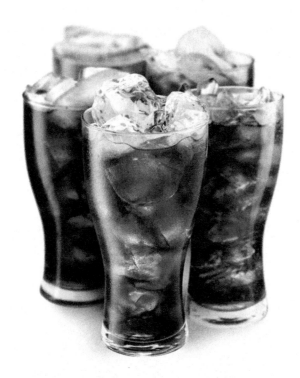

Chapter 10
Take the "Die" Out of Your Diet

Artificial sweeteners are lethal. Over time they are silent killers! Have no doubt in your mind whatsoever. Seriously, change your ways now. Drink something natural from this earth, but not rat poison! Anything but this concoction the chemists came up with to leave real sugar out of the equation. They don't care about you and I. Trust me on this. You're better off with the empty calories from the sugar than mutated genes. It's as simple as that. Diet drinks are lethal injections. Read the labels; know the killers. America drinks over nine hundred million liters of toxins a year. That's quite a few boatloads of rat poison for your guts.

Did you know that big name brand diet sodas in Ireland were recently withdrawn from the market by their manufacturers after testing positive for the presence of benzene, a cancer-causing chemical. What do you think that slippery, weird and bland aftertaste is ,that's the chemical that just took that old bitter taste and magically changed it into a sweet taste, to trick your body into ingesting it and wanting more. Put up your guard! Stop eating sugar substitutes. Your cells want to be normal, and live a long time, just like your siblings, your children, your friends, and the people who drink diet drinks all day. *Hmmm ... still want to dump in that chemical flavoring?*

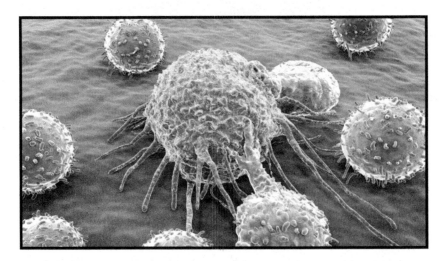

Artificial Sweeteners Cause IBS and Cancer

A sugar substitute or artificial sweetener is a food additive that attempts to duplicate the effect of sugar or corn syrup in taste, but often with less food energy. An important class of sugar substitutes are known as high intensity sweeteners. These are compounds whose sweetness is many times that of sucrose—up to hundreds of times as sweet. The sensation of sweetness caused by these compounds has a notably different mouth feel, if you've noticed. It's kind of slippery, and leaves a bitter aftertaste. That's the compound, the synthetic part, and that's what your body will try to fight off, if it can. In the U.S., five artificially derived sugar substitutes have been approved for use.

They are saccharin, aspartame, sucralose, neotame and acesulfame potassium. These compounds are all high intensity sweeteners. Studies show that they cause disease in laboratory rats. Remember what that means. The FDA determined in 1981 that aspartame was safe to use in foods, but only after it was denied for many, many years. Realizing just how much money could be made, an industry friendly director was placed in power immediately after Ronald Reagan's election

Splenda Essentials, the latest marketing venture from the makers of *Splenda,* includes vitamins, amino acids, and sometimes even fiber. The half real, half synthetic sweetener now sounds like it might actually be a healthy choice, but if a company sprinkled vitamin C on toothpaste, or added some vitamin K to mint flavored mouthwash, would you swallow it when you were done cleansing your teeth and gums?

The new *Splenda Essentials* cleverly adds vitamin B and antioxidants to its core ingredient sucralose, a nonnutritive sweetener that does not grow in sugar fields, nor does it appear naturally anywhere else on earth. Instead, sucralose is manufactured in laboratories as a synthetic compound. In other words, although *Splenda* is derived from sugar, at some point during the manufacturing process, the sugar disappears, and what remains are chlorinated atoms that are bulked up with dextrose and maltodextrin.

In a courtroom in 2007, in a bitter battle over *sweetness*, the manufacturer of *Equal* contended that the maker of *Splenda,* was misleading millions of consumers by fostering the notion, through advertising, that *Splenda* is a natural product. But the *Splenda* company argued that, "The sweetening ingredient in *Splenda* is made by a process that starts with cane sugar." It then added that, "*Splenda* is an artificial sweetener that does not contain sugar," acknowledging that the sugar disappears during the manufacturing process.

Splenda was initially marketed with the tagline, "Made from sugar, so it tastes like sugar. But it's not sugar." Then, after disappointing sales figures posted, they dropped the last sentence, and sales went through the roof.

In court, if you tell the judge half of the truth, and purposely omit facts, you can be convicted of perjury and deception, but when it comes to advertising and marketing products in the U.S., there is an enormous gray area that companies can traverse and get away with murder, or in this case, mixing a complex chemical compound with vitamins and selling it as a *healthy* sugar substitute.

Another deceiving aspect of the massively popular synthetic sweetener is that the core ingredient's name is sucralose, which is two letters fatter than sucrose, the organic compound commonly known as table sugar. On top of everything else confusing, the FDA has no real standard set for the terms *all natural*, so there are no defined parameters in place in order for a manufacturer to claim any product is truly all natural. Despite its use of sugar as the starting point for making sucralose, in no place do the words *sugar* or *sucrose* appear on Splenda's ingredients list. That is because under FDA regulations, a company cannot list a substance that has vaporized during the manufacturing process.

Sucralose is produced by substituting three chlorine atoms for three hydroxyl groups. Sucralose is not approved for use in most European countries, where national healthcare programs are prominent. Go figure. So then what is the big deal with ingesting synthetic food agents? The mother company of *Splenda*, Johnson & Johnson, contends that sucralose passes through the body unabsorbed, yet according to the FDA's *Final Rule* report, eleven to twenty seven percent of sucralose is absorbed in humans, and the rest is excreted. The Japanese Food Sanitation Council reports that up to forty percent of ingested sucralose is absorbed and can concentrate in the liver, kidney, and gastrointestinal tract, having a negative impact on overall health.

Dr. James Bowen, a biochemist and survivor of aspartame

poisoning, warns the general public about *Splenda*, saying, "Sucralose is simply chlorinated sugar." Bowen's research also reveals that sucralose can shrink thymus glands, the biological seat of immunity, and produce liver inflammation in rats and mice.

A study conducted on rats by researchers at Duke University, one of the world's foremost patient care and research institutions, determined that *Splenda* actually contributes to obesity, destroys good intestinal bacteria, and can prevent prescription drugs from being absorbed. Since real sugar is only fifteen calories per teaspoon, maybe everyone trying to manage their weight should just use the real thing in their coffee or tea. Then it would also be healthier to take the stairs instead of the elevator, park farther away from their destination and walk it off, and buy vitamins from a local health food store.

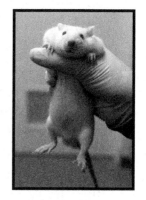

http://www.naturalnews.com/033914_Splenda_Essentials_sweetener.html#ixzz2la002bYp

Does Aspartame "preserve" dead bodies?

Aspartame is best known by the brand names *NutraSweet, Equal, Sweet One and Spoonful*. Aspartame is a synthetic chemical combination, which is comprised of approximately fifty percent phenylalanine, forty percent aspartic acid, and ten percent methanol. Aspartame is found in thousands of foods, drinks, candy, gum, vitamins, health supplements and even pharmaceuticals.

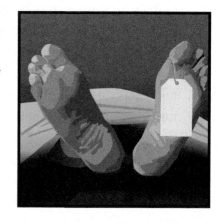

Each of the three ingredients in Aspartame poses its own dangers and each is well documented as

causing a long list of side effects and dangerous health conditions. Watch for the ingredient acesulfame potassium, which is just another name for aspartame.

Phenylalanine: Even a single use of aspartame raises the blood phenylalanine levels. High blood phenylalanine can be concentrated in parts of the brain and is especially dangerous for infants and fetuses. Because it is metabolized much more efficiently by rodents than humans, testing and research on rats alone is not sufficient enough to denounce the dangers of aspartame for human consumption. Excessive levels of phenylalanine in the brain cause serotonin levels to decrease, leading to emotional disorders like depression.

Aspartic Acid: Aspartic acid is considered an excito-toxin, which means it over stimulates certain neurons in the body until they die. Much like nitrates and MSG, aspartic acid can cause amino acid imbalances in the body and result in the interruption of normal neurotransmitter metabolism of the brain.

Methanol becomes formaldehyde (embalming fluid): The most prominent danger of aspartame is that when ingested, the methanol (wood alcohol) is distributed throughout the body, including the brain, muscle, fat and nervous tissues, and is then metabolized to form formaldehyde, which enters cells and binds to proteins and genetic material (DNA). Methanol is a dangerous neurotoxin and a known carcinogen, which causes retinal damage in the eye, interferes with DNA processes, and can cause birth defects. The EPA's recommended limit of consumption of methanol is 7.8 milligrams per day, but a one liter bottle of an Aspartame-sweetened beverage contains over 50 mg of methanol. Heavy users of Aspartame-containing products consume as much as 250 mg of methanol daily, which is over thirty times the EPA limit.

Suspiciously similar to the symptoms of fibromyalgia and multiple sclerosis, aspartame's long list includes dizziness, headaches, behavioral changes, hallucinations, depression, nausea, numbness, muscle spasms, weight gain, rashes, fatigue, irritability, insomnia, vision problems, hearing loss, heart palpitations, breathing difficulties, anxiety attacks, slurred speech, loss of taste, tinnitus, vertigo, memory loss, and joint pain. Also, many illnesses can be worsened by ingesting aspartame, including chronic fatigue syndrome, brain tumors, epilepsy, Parkinson's, Alzheimer's, mental retardation, and especially diabetes.

Birth defects: According to Dr. Louis Elsas, pediatrician professor of genetics at Emory University, phenylalanine can concentrate in the placenta, causing mental retardation of a fetus. Also, formaldehyde in the blood stream of a pregnant woman can cause her immune system to target the fetal tissue as a foreign substance and destroy it, the result being a miscarriage. This can happen before she even knows she is pregnant. (http://www.dorway.com/dr-elsas.txt)

Aspartame is known to cause weight gain

Products labeled *Diet, Light* or *Zero* most likely contain at least one of the major synthetic sweeteners, and **a**spartame is used more widely than the three carcinogenic S's: sucralose, sorbitol and saccharin. Nearly all diet sodas, gum and most candy (not chocolate—yet) are loaded with aspartame. Some chewing gum brands contain only synthetic sugars, which are acid creating. The body in turn creates fat cells to store that extra acid, and this is why many people who consistently eat Aspartame will ironically put on weight.

Natural sugar-free alternatives: Xylitol and the Brazilian *Stevia* leaf (*Not Truvia*) are natural and do not cause side effects or nerve damage; however, truly effective weight loss starts with organic vegetables and cardio exercise. To be safe, simply avoid all diet foods and moderate sugar intake.

http://www.naturalnews.com/034320_aspartame_sweetener_side_effects.html#ixzz2la1qTVwP

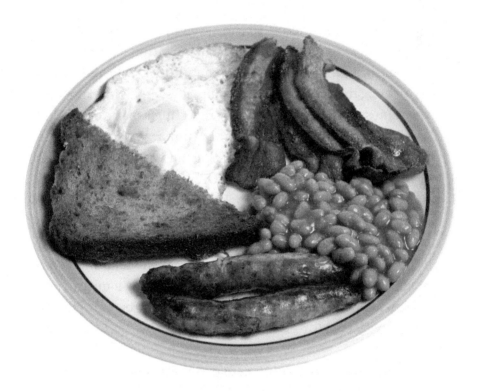

Chapter 11
Fried food

One of our favorite foods may be among the worst for us: fried chicken boiled in vats of grease and oils. Fried chicken batter is often basically flour, sugar, salt, black pepper and monosodium glutamate (MSG). The problem is with the entire recipe! When one fries the chicken pieces dipped in this batter at high temperatures, it leads to the creation of acrylamides, toxic chemical by-products of cooking that are believed by many health experts to promote cancer. In fact, as per one scientific study, eating acrylamides boosts kidney cancer rates by nearly sixty percent. It is also linked to ovarian cancer.

Why are fried foods terrible for your health?

Fried foods damage your body and brain in many different ways, and it's not just a long term consequence, but a short term detriment as well. Just as a car needs good clean oil to run efficiently and not break down, your body needs food that can be digested properly and not clog the one and only machine you have for your entire life. You simply can't lie to yourself much with fried food because the ill effects are just too obvious. Simply grab some belly fat or pinch an inch on a hip or thigh, and then try to convince yourself it's okay. Plus, obesity basically means people are storing fried foods and carbohydrates as body fat, and for about a third of Americans, it's like carry-on luggage you can't set down, or at least not until you sit down.

Face the fried food facts:

- Fried foods clog arteries and lead to strokes and Alzeimer's.
- Clogged veins and arteries cause heart attacks and aneurysms.
- Canola oil is one of the top 3 GMO products (genetically modified to contain pesticides) in U.S. and is used by almost all restaurants and for nearly all fried products you find in stores.
- Canola oil (rapeseed oil) is synthetic and deprives cells of oxygen, causing emphysema and respiratory distress, eventually leading to cancer.
- Soy and soy by-products are almost all GMO.
- Corn oil and corn by-products (breading on almost everything) are also GMO and contain pesticide (http://breathing. com/articles/canola-oil.htm).
- Most fried foods contain MSG (toxic salts) to enhance "dead food" flavor
- Taking antacids makes things worse, preventing natural enzyme production by the body. It also adds bad calcium which is armor (protection) for parasites/infection.
- Most meats are from animals, fowl and "farm raised" fish that are loaded with hormones and antibiotics.

- Fried means inflammatory foods which create problems with joints.
- Arterial plaque increases blood pressure.
- Potatoes and most bread (buns/pizza crust/pitas/tortillas, etc.) soak up the canola oil and turn to sugar in the stomach.
- Modified, processed and fried foods don't break down in body properly; remaining in kidneys, liver, intestines, prostate and colon for extended periods of time, if not forever.
- Gluten (mutant food glue): Used for pizza crust, fried seafood, pre-prepped Chinese, corn dogs, crackers, pastries, cakes, and the list is a mile long.
- Sugar and carbs feed infection; makes you want more of the same; feeding the vicious cycle.
- Empty calories are totally void of nutrients, so the body keeps searching for anything of nutritional value. Plus, the "full" feeling wears off sooner, leading to overeating.

Clogged drains and veins

Here's a hard truth perspective: Eating fried chicken and pan pizza cooked in GMO oil is one of the worst things you can do to your body. Basically, fried food breading soaks up nearly every drop of the canola oil, so eating fried chicken and pan pizza is like drinking oil straight from the vat. This increases your low-density or "bad" cholesterol. The inner portion of your arteries is meant to be smooth and unrestricted, but the buildup from these saturated fats, cholesterol and trans-fats can cause hard deposits (plaque) to form. Then, like a clog in a drain, your blood flow can become completely blocked and result in a heart attack or stroke, especially if a piece of the plaque breaks away.

Also, *the closer your fat is to your heart, the more the heart is strained.* It's worse for men because the belly is closer to the heart than the hips and thighs, where women are more prone to keep the fried foods "stored." That is one reason women have a longer life span than men on average.

The great news is that *you can unclog your arteries without surgery or drugs*. If you've been binging on fried foods, you need to detoxify your blood and refortify organs. Take plenty of organic B vitamins, and check into dandelion root and milk thistle. Periodic detoxification is like changing the oil in your car; it must be done.

Look online and find your local vitamin shop and health food stores. You must plan and prepare healthy meals, so when you have a hunger attack you won't cave in. Get creative! Want to fry some foods at home so you don't feel left out? Dip your favorite vegetables in organic eggs and then roll them in organic bread crumbs. In about a quarter inch of olive oil, slightly brown one side and then flip them over. Artichokes can replace those fried shrimp and oysters and mushrooms replace fries! Try it.

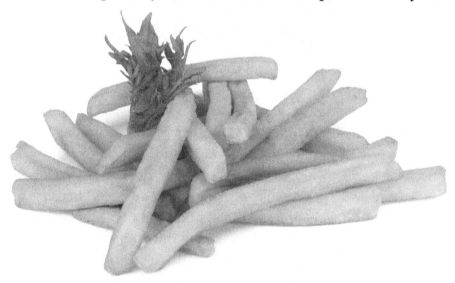

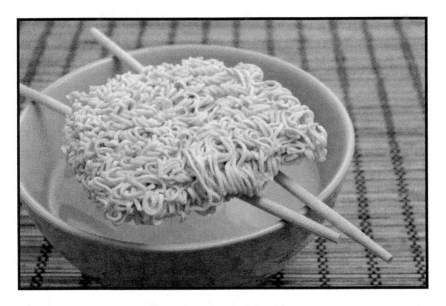

Chapter 12
MSG

Monosodium Glutamate, better known as MSG, is a form of concentrated salt added to foods to enhance the flavor. This salt version of glutamic acid is an amino acid the body can produce on its own, but the MSG we find on store shelves is processed and comes from fermented *sugar beets*. Because this kind of MSG is processed, it can cause many adverse reactions, including skin rashes, itching, hives, nausea, vomiting, migraine headaches, asthma, heart irregularities, depression and even seizures. http://www.msgtruth.org/migraine.htm

Since MSG acquired its infamous reputation for causing migraines, the food industry has given it *new names and new forms*, including autolyzed yeast, yeast extract, maltodextrin, hydrolyzed protein, sodium caseinate, mono-potassium glutamate, and textured protein. Consumers who are watching out for monosodium glutamate in long ingredients lists usually don't know the aliases, but should.

Because MSG is so cheap, the food industry can use much lower quality foods and simply add MSG as a flavor enhancer. Currently, there is a huge investment by the food giants in MSG medical research to convince consumers of its safety. MSG contains the gene of the pesticide *Roundup*. Consumers who don't filter MSG out of their diet are catching a double dose of toxicity.

Foods which contain the largest doses of MSG are spicy corn chips, many soups, certain Chinese foods, ranch dressing, sausages, hot dogs, barbecued meats, smoked meats, processed deli meats, and sauces. Also included are most powdered packets like chili, gravy, taco seasoning, French onion dip and dried dip mixes.

Ibuprofen is the polar opposite of MSG. This widely used painkiller is specifically designed to relieve symptoms from MSG headaches, but only temporarily. Unfortunately, most research on MSG is done by its manufacturers in independent labs. The FDA itself consists of food industry reps and lobbyists who help keep MSG approved, so most doctors (except naturopath doctors) will not point their finger at MSG as the cause of headaches, inflammation, weight gain, muscle pain, or nerve disorders.

MSG affects the central nervous system

Consuming products loaded with MSG on an empty stomach or without water can be especially dangerous. MSG affects nearly everyone because it causes a spike in glutamic acid, which is used throughout the body as a neurotransmitter, so many migraines are accompanied by photo-sensitivity (sensitivity to light) and phono-sensitivity (sensitivity to sound). This explains why many people need to relax in a dark, quiet room to recover. MSG compromises the way the liver and gall bladder use bile to break up fats for digestion, so many people experience diarrhea and even gall bladder attacks. Others will vomit or stir up their Irritable Bowel Syndrome.

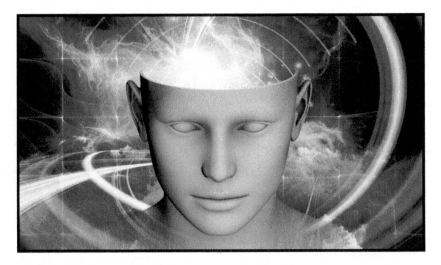

Also, the hair cells of the ear use glutamate as a neurotransmitter, so over stimulation of these cells can result in ringing in the ears (also tinnitus or vertigo). MSG is known to cross the blood brain barrier to damage brain cells, especially in infants. Research has also shown that MSG can cause sterility in female animals. Since there are no *regulations on the potency of MSG,* consumers have no way of knowing how much or how little they are getting. Plus, the sooner MSG appears in an ingredients list, the more there is in that product. Consuming MSG at any time is a risk many consumers are not willing to take. There are several reliable sources on this:

http://www.vanderbilt.edu/ans/psychology/hea...

http://www.msgtruth.org/migraine.htm

http://www.naturalnews.com/034272_MSG_monosodium_glutamate.html#ixzz2pRdYJ09H

Your best bet is to avoid MSG in general and just add your own natural spices to foods. Sea salt and fresh garlic or organic minced garlic can give a dish the same taste and flavor enhancement. Simply Tasteful's "Garlic Garlic" or "Onion Onion" and Trader Joe's "21 Seasoning Salute" are great natural seasonings that take food flavor up a notch and don't cause headaches, nausea or nerve damage.

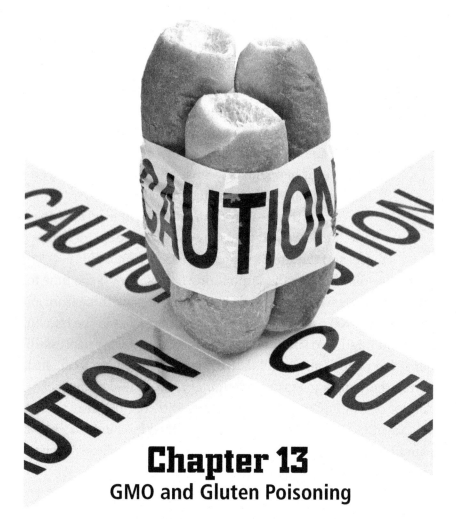

Chapter 13
GMO and Gluten Poisoning

Let's delve into how genetically modified food and gluten (pesticide food glue) ruin lives by wrecking the general health of millions, including children and babies.

Believe it or not, most depression comes from what we eat. Think of how most chickens, pigs and cows are treated by the monster corporations that control and manipulate the breeding grounds on many of our country's farms, and you will get a good idea of the definition of depression. For most of the masses, the poor animals do not live a normal farm life. They're cooped up in small pens like prisons, over populated and unkempt, in quarters full of their own feces and unable to roam as healthy animals do normally. They're separated from their mothers shortly after birth. This is the horror of a processed life undeserved by God's animals, which includes being shot up with estrogen hormones and antibiotics, to make them meatier and kill the bacteria all at the same time. We eat the meat of these corporate prisoners, after they lead a life of pure depression, and we serve them on our dinner table, and we order them in drive-through windows, like it never happened, because we didn't see it happen, and hardly anybody is facing up to the reality.

You eat the meat from an animal that lived its whole, short life depressed. And now you go to the doctor and get advice, and the latest version of *Prozac, Xanax, lithium*; all the while still following the same eating habits. Now is the time to stop wondering why you're so depressed. Eating anything from an animal that lived a depressed life fosters depression in the human body and mind, and since you are what you eat, you are depressed. For some people, almost all they eat is chemical laden food. Just saying the names makes people hungry, but it makes me sick. I am not one of Pavlov's dogs salivating. Did you just hear a bell? Just say no to GMO! The genetically modified food industry has a plan for the negligent, the lazy—the junk science addicts. America makes it so viable for the masses to eat depressed meat.

Pesticides

Bug killer and weed killer make corporate driven farmers more money, or at least it used to, but now thanks to *Superbugs* and *Superweeds*, conventional farming uses more and more bug killer and weed killer on their crops, and they are buying seeds which contain these same bug and weed killer formulas in their DNA, so when you eat that food, your body can now create that pesticide. This is what people don't understand and have never heard about, and this is what is killing Americans faster than anything else on the planet.

The farmers who sellout to Biotech companies like Monsanto, Dupont, Bayer, and Dow Chemical, agree on contract to ex-

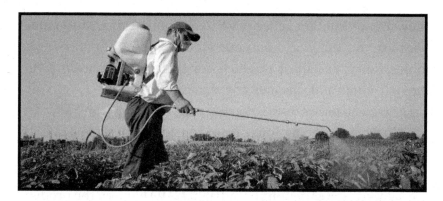

clusively use these lethal pesticides and GM seeds, and they are locked into an evil agricultural nightmare. Over the past twenty years of this genetically modified farming practice, beetles, worms, caterpillars and all kinds of weeds have grown immune to mainly Monsanto's *RoundUp* chemical combo, and their BT corn and now over seventy-five percent of conventional food is loaded with such a heavy dose of cancer chemicals that the human body just can't beat back anymore. People consuming GMO food on a regular basis can expect cancer cells to move in for the kill in just a couple of decades now, if not sooner.

There are molecular engineers working right now in laboratories for Monsanto, gene-splicing vegetable seedlings with pesticides and herbicides so the plants are better protected from the insects and worms that might damage them.

What happens to the brain, the heart, the central nervous system, and the livers of the humans that consume bug and weed killer on a regular basis? What happens to the cells and the immunity system of the human *bugs* that are eating GMO? Do you have IBS? Do you have a weak liver? Do you have cancer? The cold fact is that the majority of products Americans eat daily contain some form of GMO soy, corn, canola (rapeseed) oil or cotton seed oil. Research shows that consuming the popular herbicide *Roundup* leads to mutation of cells thus fueling the development of malignant tumors and other various forms of cancer. In other words, as the plants grow up from the ground, they already contain genes from toxic concoctions. Most countries around the world ban our GMO exports of major vegetables, dairy, and meat products for this specific reason. Even most flu shots and vaccines now contain GMO.

http://www.naturalnews.com/034209_GMOs_questions.html#ixzz2aM9iMJhq

Most developed nations do not consider GMOs to be safe. In more than sixty countries around the world, including Australia, Japan, and all of the countries in the European Union, there are significant restrictions or outright GMO bans on the production and sale and/or import of genetically "mutated" food. In the U.S., the government has approved GMOs based on studies conducted by the same corporations that created them and profit from their sale. How ridiculous is that? That would be like letting stock brokers oversee all inside trading activity. Increasingly, Americans are taking matters into their own hands and choosing to opt out of the GMO experiment.

One of the most widely used, and well known, GMOs is gluten, which is used to bulk up food. All wheat, rye and barley contain gluten, whether GMO or not. It's used as a thickening agent and filler in everything from biscuits and bread to crackers and cereals. The inactive ingredients in many medications are gluten-based. And even when gluten isn't an ingredient, it may inadvertently get into a food because a wheat-based food was processed in the same factory, or wheat was grown in a nearby field. Also, most of the animal feed given to CAFO animals contains GMO and gluten, so the "feed" are given toxic feed. Its a vicious cycle.

It should be spelled **glue—ton** because it's like a ton of glue food stuck to your insides, that contains synthetic ingredients including pesticide, insecticide, herbicide, fungicide, DNA from other organisms including insects, and processed ingredients. These substances rot in your intestines and wreak havoc on your digestive system and your filtering organs. Your liver, kidneys, pancreas are necessary for your survival. It's time to wake up and filter out the toxic *glue food* from your intake.

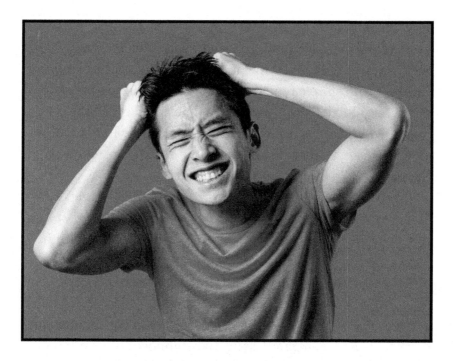

Chapter 14
Signs of Stress

Just as your car or truck needs clean gas, clean oil, and a clean air filter to function properly, your body needs "clean" food. If you pour in the wrong kind of oil, or gas that's loaded with "fillers" or your exhaust system is clogged up, your car will give you obvious and immediate signs of system breakdown, like bucking when you step on the gas, or smoke coming out of the tail pipe, or the "check engine" light will come on. What will you do about it?

Will you pour in more dirty gas and more of the wrong oil? Will you try to keep driving until the engine completely fails? Will you drive to the first car doctor (rip-off mechanic) and get the latest prescription (car parts or "diagnostic" you don't need) and waste your money, your time, and destroy all common sense when it comes to proper maintenance? What ever happened to preventive maintenance?

It's time to understand that your symptoms are simply your body's way of telling you to check fluid. All of those symptoms are signs with simple remedies that will provide you with a long lasting, productive engine (the only one you'll ever have). That engine will burn clean fuel, it will fire on all cylinders all the time, and won't break down when you need it most, and that's every day.

Without further ado, here are eight telltale signs that you've consumed some toxic food and your *symptoms* need more than just cover up medicine:

1. You have a migraine headache: Most headaches are the result of dehydration. Drink only natural spring water and stop consuming concentrated salts like monosodium glutamate (MSG), hydrolyzed soy protein, autolyzed yeast extract and maltodextrin. Also, never drink water from the tap, as it contains fluoride and bleach, which add to dehydration and other chronic health problems.

2. You are experiencing inflammation or edema: Are you retaining abnormal amounts of water? This could show up as weight gain. Do your hands and feet swell often? Are you consuming excessive animal protein, dairy, or GM wheat? What about refined sugars? Check the sodium levels in processed foods, especially ones you ate in the past 6 hours. Most doctors will not tell you that this is a dietary problem.

3. You have vertigo (dizziness): This is usually an equilibrium issue in the inner ear, boiling right back to diet. Check your recent intake for MSG, Aspartame, nitrates in meats and concentrated sweets. (http://www.drfuhrman.com)

4. You are constipated or you have diarrhea, stomach pains, acid reflux or irritable bowels (IBS): Gluten is "mutant" GMO food "glue" and causes constipation. Gluten and artificial sweeteners can irritate your entire digestive tract and pollute your cleansing organs with synthetic toxins which may never release. Your body knows when you've consumed these "poisons" and lets you know right away. Pay attention to the warning signs.

5. You are breaking out with a skin rash, eczema or psoriasis: Check your concentrated sweets, gluten, GMO pesticide-laden foods like corn and soy, and remember, the more processed food you eat, the more you break out with these skin conditions. Even typical medications like aspirin, cough syrup and ibuprofen can be overdone and cause headaches and rashes.

6. You are experiencing lethargy: Nothing slows down a human body faster than "trash" food. Any athlete will tell you "garbage in - garbage out," which means if you eat nutrient-void food, you will not have any energy. It's not complicated. Read more about organic food and Superfoods and realize you don't have to reinvent the wheel to get rolling on the highway of vitality. (http://www.mybitesofbliss.com/)

7. You are caught in a massive brain fog: Did you just drink some tap water? Did you just get a flu shot or a vaccine? Did you just eat something with aspartame in it? Did you just return from the dentist with a new mercury cavity filling? Did you just take some toxic pharmaceutical medication for anxiety, depression or ADHD? Visit the Health Ranger's Nutrition Store on line for the natural remedy: (http://store.naturalnews.com)

8. You have no motivation and you are depressed: Everyone has heard the saying, "You are what you eat." It's true. If you eat animals that lived their whole life depressed, you will experience depression. If you eat pesticide and insecticide that makes bugs sick, you will be sick. Know what's in your food at all times. Get the free phone app called "Fooducate" and scan the barcodes of every food product for toxins, before you buy anything! (http://www.fooducate.com/)

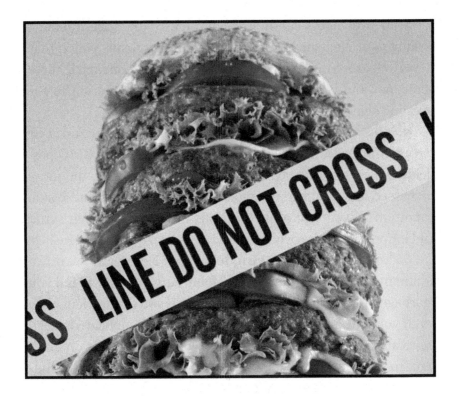

Chapter 15
16 Food Filtering Tips

Let's take a look at "junk science" and the temptations that lead to malfunctions, of the digestive tract, of the alkalinity of your blood, and of how much oxygen your cells receive. Look at the body as a whole and its functions as holistic. Here are some common foods to avoid like the plague, and your body will reward you with energy, vitality, and overall good health. This is Health Basics 101, and you can use it as a template for which foods to avoid, and also for finding foods you love that are good for you and rewarding.

■ Fried foods clog arteries and lead to strokes and Alzheimer's.
■ Clogged veins and arteries cause heart attacks and aneurysms.

- Canola oil is one of the top 3 GMO products (genetically modified to contain pesticides) in U.S. and is used by almost all restaurants and for nearly all fried products you find in stores.
- Canola oil (rapeseed oil) is synthetic and deprives cells of oxygen, causing emphysema and respiratory distress, eventually leading to cancer.
- Soy and soy by-products are almost all GMO.
- Corn oil and corn by-products (breading on almost everything) are also GMO and contain pesticide (http://breathing.com/articles/canola-oil.htm).
- Most fried foods contain MSG (toxic salts) to enhance "dead food" flavor
- Taking antacids makes things worse—prevents natural enzyme production by the body. It also adds bad calcium which is armor (protection) for parasites/infection.
- Most meats are from animals, fowl and "farm raised" fish that are loaded with hormones and antibiotics.
- Fried means inflammatory foods which create problems with joints.
- Arterial plaque increases blood pressure.
- Potatoes and most bread (buns/pizza crust/pitas/tortillas, etc.) soak up the canola oil and turn to sugar in the stomach.
- Modified, processed and fried foods don't break down in body properly; remaining in kidneys, liver, intestines, prostate and colon for extended periods of time, if not forever.
- Gluten (mutant food glue): Used for pizza crust, fried seafood, pre-prepped Chinese, corn dogs, crackers, pastries, cakes, and the list is a mile long.
- Sugar and carbohydrates feed infection; makes you want more of the same; feeding the vicious cycle.
- Empty calories are totally void of nutrients, so the body stays hungry, searching for nutrients. Also, the feeling of being full wears off sooner and hunger for "junk science food" returns.

http://www.naturalnews.com/034483_fried_foods_health_damage.html

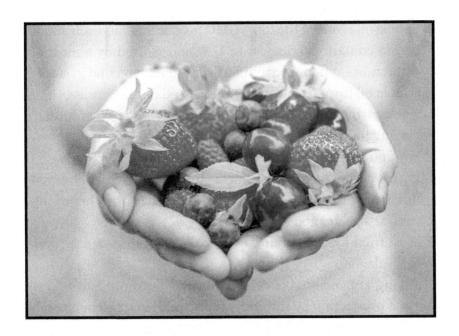

Chapter 16
Organic and Kosher

Are you confused about food label claims and what they really mean? That's part of the strategy of the global food giants, of course, to confuse you with so much noise that you give up trying to make sense of it all. *The Health Ranger,* Mike Adams, is a nutritionist and scientist who demystified food label claims for us very well, and many of the following points will probably surprise you. Here are the top tweleve misunderstandings summarized for your convenience:

1. "Kosher" does not mean non-GMO
Genetically engineered ingredients are openly allowed in Kosher-certified foods. The Kosher certification does not involve testing for GMOs, and Kosher certifications are routinely found on foods containing GMOs. Additives like MSG are allowed, and MSG is certainly GMO.

2. "Organic" does not mean low in heavy metals

The USDA certified organic certification process does not test for heavy metals. Foods that are very high in lead, arsenic, cadmium, mercury and even aluminum are openly allowed to be labeled USDA certified organic.

3. "Non-GMO" does not mean organic

Just because a food is certified non-GMO doesn't mean it is organic. Even conventionally-raised crops such as corn, soy and canola can be certified non-GMO if they are grown without genetically engineered seeds. There are several snack chips on the market right now that use non-GMO ingredients grown with chemical pesticides.

4. "All Natural" doesn't mean anything at all

The phrase "All Natural" is not regulated in any way by the FDA. Any foods, including foods made with artificial colors, chemical sweeteners, chemical preservatives and GMOs, can be labeled "all natural." "All natural" is the trick used by large food corporations to try to mislead consumers into thinking their junk food products are somehow organic.

5. "Trans-Fat Free" does not mean free from trans fats

The FDA currently allows foods containing up to 0.5g of trans fats per serving to claim ZERO grams of trans fats per serving. Can you believe it? Big food and drug corporations have convinced the FDA to allow food labels to blatantly lie to consumers about what the food really contains. Everywhere else in the world, 0.5 does not equal zero. Even in high school math class, it's rounded up to one. But at the FDA, 0.5 somehow means zero. What if you were allergic to penicillin and your medicine said penicillin-free, but still contained .5 percent – you could die! Maybe you won't die from a little trans-fat, but still, it's just not right.

6. "Non-GMO" does not mean certified non-GMO

There are many foods, superfoods and even nutritional products currently claiming to be "non-GMO" but failing to provide any certification of that status. A company that self-proclaims its products to be "non-GMO" is most likely trying to pull a fast one on you unless it can back up that claim with certification. Only **certified non-GMO** means something. The next time you see a label that claims "non-GMO," ask yourself, "Certified by whom?" "Where's the proof?"

7. "Gluten-free" foods are often GMO

Beware of GMOs in gluten-free foods. Gluten-free foods are usually made with genetically modified corn containing *BT toxin*, a deadly insecticide. Avoid gluten-free unless it's also certified non-GMO.

8. "Organic" foods can still contain a small amount of GMO

GMOs are so widespread that they have now contaminated virtually the entire food supply. Foods that are certified organic can still contain trace levels of GMOs. How much are they allowed to contain? There aren't specific tolerance levels in the USDA organic regulations for GMOs. However, even though certified organic foods can still contain trace levels of GMOs, they are still far healthier for you than conventionally-grown foods!

9. "Organic" foods are now being routinely grown in heavily polluted countries such as China

An increasing percentage of "organic" foods, superfoods and raw materials used in nutritional supplements are being imported from China. *Natural News* has found that these raw materials are consistently higher in heavy metals than competing products grown in North America. Watch out, my friends. Organic certification standards openly allow organic farms in China to grow produce in fields that are heavily polluted with cadmium, lead and mercury. There is no limit on the heavy metals levels in soils used to produce USDA certified organic foods.

10. The FDA currently has no limit on the amount of heavy metals allowed in foods, either

The FDA does not publish or set any official limits on heavy metals in imported foods. Usually, when the FDA does find metals in foods they denounce them by blatantly ignoring the long-term health risks. Basically, as long as the food is dead and not carrying e.coli or salmonella, there is almost no food too polluted for the FDA to approve.

11. The use of "organic" ingredients does not automatically make the whole product organic

Some products sold today are being described as "organic" when only a fraction of their ingredients are organic. This does not qualify a product to be called organic. Unlike the phrase, "all natural," the term "organic" is highly regulated by the federal government and carries a specific meaning.

12. "Low calorie" almost always means it is sweetened with a chemical sweetener

Look on the ingredients labels of "low calorie" foods or beverages, and you'll almost always find sucralose, acesulfame potassium, saccharin, aspartame or other chemical sweeteners. Anything with the name or slogan "low calorie," "light," or "zero" is a huge red flag!

Is it Kosher?

For some, meat is a must. They just don't want to give it up totally. So to those who stay that route, look for *organic* meat and *kosher* symbols. Kosher: what does it mean, and why is it better for the meats we eat?

There is no question that some of the kosher dietary laws have beneficial health effects. The laws regarding kosher slaughter are so sanitary that kosher butchers and slaughterhouses have been exempted from many USDA regulations. The method of slaughter is a quick, deep stroke across the throat with a perfectly sharp blade with no nicks or unevenness. A trained kosher slaughterer, or shochet, severs the trachea and esophagus of the animal with a special razor-sharp knife. This also severs the jugular vein, causing near-instantaneous death with minimal pain to the animal.

This method causes unconsciousness within two seconds, and is widely recognized as the most humane method of slaughter possible. Another advantage is that it ensures rapid, complete draining of the blood, which is also necessary to render the meat kosher. With its extra supervision, kosher food is perceived as being healthier and cleaner. After slaughter, animals are checked for abscesses in their lungs or other health problems. Blood, an easy medium for the growth of bacteria, is drained.

Do "Organic" and "Kosher" labels still matter?

Absolutely they matter. For example, raw organic virgin coconut oil has a hundred uses for health and home. Kosher meats come from animals that were treated much more humanely, which means that meat will tax your system less.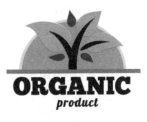

Many health-conscious people have decided to refrain from eating meat. Additionally, many humane-conscious people have eliminated meat from their diet. Both groups have good reasons for their decisions.

Kosher meats are those listed in the Bible as derived from animals deemed edible for the Jewish people. Any animal with a cloven hoof that chews its cud is allowable; conversely, those which lack both of these characteristics are forbidden. Cattle, sheep, and goats are examples of kosher mammals. Horses, dogs and pigs are forbidden. Birds are allowable according to custom, but generally, it seems that birds of prey are forbidden. Chicken, quail, and doves are kosher; *eagles are forbidden*.

Keeping kosher also has to do with the way the animal is slaughtered. The Bible is clear in its instruction that Jews are not to eat the animal's blood. It is also taught that man is not to cause the suffering of any other living thing. As a result, from the time of the giving of the instructions, a procedure has been carried down through the generations detailing how the throat is to be cut and the blood drained immediately. The cut is to be swift and sure, done with a knife that is always to be kept sharp and free of nicks. Done correctly, a kosher slaughter causes very little or no discernible suffering to the animal.

Unfortunately, in recent months there have been instances at one large kosher slaughterhouse in which humane treatment has been lacking. Also, some kosher meat is imported from South America, in which less than humane procedures might be used. For these reasons, consumers should check on the origin of the meat he or she is considering purchasing. The kosher slaughtering procedure has been shown to have direct results on meat quality. Plus, the bleeding out of the kosher slaughtered animal provides an additional protection against potentially infectious organisms which are generally transmitted in the blood.

Humane treatment of animals makes for healthier food

The humane treatment of animals is important on a nutritional level. Research has shown that there appears to be a fear pheromone released in the blood by animals undergoing stress. While many consumers have been made aware of the problems with meat from animals who have been given hormones, most are not aware that hormones also enter the meat naturally through the bloodstreams of stressed, fearful and hurt animals. Consider this: Fear experienced during the *slaughtering process* results in elevated levels of steroid hormones, generally associated with adrenal-cortical secretions. These remain in the meat and are transmitted to those who eat it. Humans have been found to be particularly susceptible to their effects. A study in Britain found the more meat eaten by pregnant mothers, the higher the levels of stress hormone, cortisol, was found in the child.

http://www.naturalnews.com/022446_kosher_meat_foods.html#ixzz2pRxBtlnF

What the heck is gelatin, really?

For decades now, gelatin has come from *abused, hormone-fed, antibiotic-injected, sick, dying and disease-laden animals.* It comes from the skin, cartilage, connective tissues, decaying hides, and the bones of those animals. Worldwide production of gelatin exceeds three hundred thousand tons per year. Vegetarian or not, everyone who takes vitamins and supplements from gelatin capsules is likely eating infected animal parts, a little bit at a time, over and over and over again.

Lard is fat from a pig's abdomen

Lard is the fat from the abdomen of a pig that is rendered and clarified for use in cooking. Nutritionists have been telling us for decades that animal fat can cause heart attacks and we should cut down on meat consumption, but what if you're eating it and you don't even know? Pig fat can clog your arteries, and when blood clots and gets stuck, blocking the artery it can cause a heart attack. Everyone knows this, right? Lard, solidified pig fat, has been considered among the worst offenders. It's time to double check the icing on your desserts and the crust of your pies. It's not hard to make your own delicious treats with organic honey, coconut oil and organic fruits. Also, check out natural sugar substitutes like xylitol and stevia.

http://ecodevoevo.blogspot.com

Chicken stock could be any part of the chicken

The cheapest chicken *parts* are used for flavoring, thickening soups and stews and for dehydrating spices and sauces.

There's no telling what part of a chicken you are eating if you're eating chicken stock, and there's no way to really check, not by looking at it, tasting it or checking for labels, especially if they don't even exist. It happens to vegans and vegetarians all the time. They forget to ask, and nobody says anything otherwise. They take a bite of some stuffed mushrooms and to their dismay they're eating chicken stock. They eat a bowl of egg drop soup or hot and sour soup, and oops, they're consuming chicken stock. And just where does all that "stock" come from? The answer is CAFOs. It all adds up, like I said earlier. Knowledge is power. Realize what is in most conventional food and I bet you will stop eating it. Think about it.

Beware of Chicken Stock

Confined animal feeding operations (CAFOs) are a complete and utter nightmarish world for animals, as they are very inhumane. As for us humans, since you are what you eat, if you eat animals that lead a depressed, unhealthy life, guess what you become? - Depressed and unhealthy. Learn more about CAFOs and about the dangers of eating chicken stock. In fact, do yourself a huge favor and start asking questions about dishes at restaurants that might contain chicken stock. Only buy supplements that are vegetarian and/or organic, and stop buying any supplements that are contained in a gelatin capsule. Phase out or get rid of gelatin capsules and buy only vegetarian! Last but not least, make your own pie crust at home, without lard, and make your own organic desserts, there are lots of creative ideas out there that are simple and delicious, and even good for you.

http://www.naturalnews.com/042830_vegetarians_restaurants_eating_dead_animals.html#ixzz2pRvzHkHL

http://www.thedailygreen.com

http://www.rawfullytempting.com

http://www.peopleforanimalsindia.org

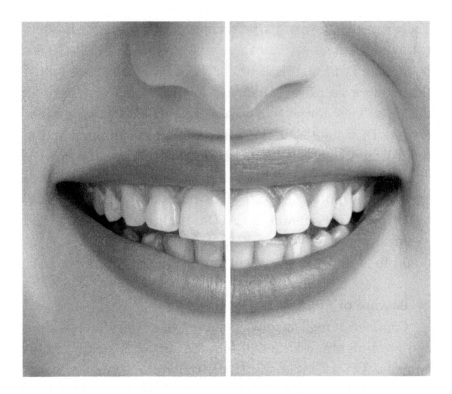

Chapter 17
Teeth Whiteners

Are you serious? Please tell me you're not drinking peroxide bleach! Oh, you just keep it in your mouth for three hours, and then spit it out, but you don't swallow any. That sounds safe! And what about the whitening strips you wear for an hour each night for a month? Or better yet, the bleach-filled mouthpiece you sleep with all night long. I'm sure your subconscious mind is conscious enough while you're sleeping to keep you from swallowing any of that bleach. That's just great.

So, let me ask you, would you drink a glass of bleach out of a dare, just to see what happens? What if I gave you one hundred dollars? Would you do it? Come on, it's not enough to give you cancer. How about just taking a teaspoon of bleach with each meal, sort of like a shot of whiskey. Guess what? You pretty much already do. Ever eat white rice (except for Basmati)? What about white sugar? And white bread? Did you forget about white pasta? What about bleached flour? Those foods are not naturally white! People think it is better food, maybe cleaner or something, because it's white. White rice, white pasta, white bread and white sugar poison you with bleach! Maybe it's time to put up your guard.

The teeth-whitening craze *is* crazy. You might as well be brushing your teeth with gasoline or bug spray. Plus, fluoride toothpaste eats away at your enamel. Plus, as you weaken your teeth, which most dentists excuse as just "sensitivity", you also damage your gums, the lining of your mouth, and your throat with one of the most toxic chemicals in the entire world.

Buy fluoride free toothpaste and you'll still have your teeth when you're one hundred years old. If every household in the U.S. replaced one bottle of 48 oz. chlorine bleach with non-chlorine bleach we could prevent more than eight million pounds of chlorine from entering our environment. Keep that stuff out of your mouth and your stomach! Don't use toothpaste with bleach, never bleach your teeth for hours in a mouthpiece, and don't chew teeth-whitening gum. Guards up!

We're awash in bleach. It's in our tap water in the form of chlorine. Don't ever drink water directly from the tap, and don't use tap water to fill up your water bottle or your juice jug for *Kool-aid* or sweet tea. Use a water purifier.

Chlorine is the greatest enabler of cancer of the bladder and prostate. Would you eat or drink something that burns when you leave it on your hands? It will burn the lining of your insides, and cancer will attack those spots first. Better yet, drink spring water. You can find a spring near you at findaspring.com.

The chemicals in tap water cause reduced growth and development, cancer, organ damage, nervous system damage, and in extreme cases, death. Exposure to some metals, such as mercury and lead, may also cause development of autoimmunity, in which a person's immune system attacks its own cells. Sound familiar? This can lead to joint diseases such as rheumatoid arthritis, and diseases of the kidneys, circulatory system, and nervous system. Kids are more prone to the toxic effects of heavy metals, as the rapidly developing body systems in the fetus, infants and young children are far more sensitive. Childhood exposure to some metals can result in learning difficulties, memory impairment, damage to the nervous system, and behavioral problems. Children may receive higher doses of metals from food than adults, since they consume more food for their body weight than adults.

If you fill a pitcher of water from the sink, just let it sit out for about twenty four hours and all the chemicals, like chlorine, will evaporate, then you don't have buy bottled water. Plus, bottled water brings with it its own dangers, like bisphenol-A.

Do certain teeth whiteners cause cancer? Well, the question isn't whether they cause cancer, but how soon will the cancerous cells in your body find the damaged tissue—tissue that has been irritated over and over and suffered for years from your peroxide ingestion. It adds up faster than you might think. I hear about tons of people in their forties dying of cancer, and most of the time the cancer attacks their cleansing organs, like the liver, spleen, or kidneys.

Teeth whiteners can and do cause cancer of the soft tissues of the mouth. That's where the cancer will start. Don't think so? Oh, the dentist told you otherwise? That's because they make a fortune from people sitting in their chairs for three hours on end, waiting for the bleach to make their teeth white.Meanwhile, the precious peroxide contained in those teeth whitener products breaks down to form molecules called free radicals. It's these free radicals that are capable of causing cellular damage. The free radicals will travel to skin tissue or an organ that's been weakened over the years, so it can attach itself and start multiplying. This is the best example of the work of mutagens, as they change your DNA for the worse.

Bisphenol A

This deadly toxin is being absorbed into bottled water from plastic containers, and the longer the water is stored, the more the levels of poison increase. Small doses can make you feel ill and depressed, and larger quantities can cause violent vomiting and even death. After testing, levels of this poison doubled when the bottles were stored for more than three months. Look for cracks or cloudiness on your reusable clear plastic bottles, don't keep your bottled water for more than a season, and you should be okay.

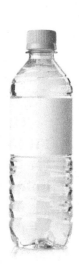

Peroxides

Free radical damage stems from the hydrogen peroxide that's in the gels we apply to whiten our teeth, and it's loaded in over-the-counter, self-application bleaching kits that whiten teeth. Many products often contain carbamide peroxide, one-third of which is composed of hydrogen peroxide. When used as a whitener, carbamide peroxide changes into hydrogen peroxide.

In animal studies, peroxide has been shown to promote the growth of cancerous tumors inside the cheeks of rodents and cause gastrointestinal cancers *when ingested.* Specifically, the theory is that when hydrogen peroxide leaks from trays containing the whitening gel onto surrounding areas inside the mouth, it triggers the release of cancer-causing free radical cells. Of course, no tests have been done on humans, except for the millions of people who are using it now and will get the results when they start chemotherapy.

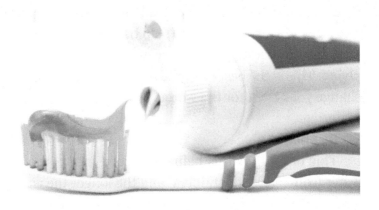

Here's a list of places where you'll find either ARTI-FICIAL SWEETENERS (rat poison) or BLEACH (pancreatic/bladder cancer) in your regularly used household products:

White coffee filters

Flour

White sugar and white rice

Tums and chewable vitamins (unbelievable!)

Nyquil (that'll put you to sleep for good).

Tylenol and Robitussin (great for the kids)

Maalox for reflux

Toothpaste and Mouthwash

Breath mints,

and of course...

Nearly all "sugar free" gum and candy

Yes, I said it! Don't chew it and don't eat it. Orbit gum lists Sorbitol as the first ingredient on the package. That means there's more of that chemical than any other ingredient in the pack. Why don't they just market Sorbitol as a treat all by itself, that way we can just ingest a pure killer without all the hype and disguises. Most sugar free gum has no natural ingredients whatsoever! You are chewing ten different chemicals that lead to fibromyalgia, nerve disorders, headaches and IBS—irritable bowel syndrome.

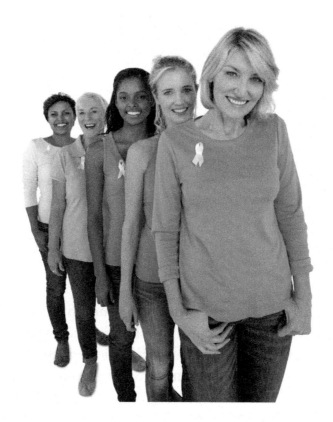

Chapter 18
Breast Cancer: Hormones and Deodorant

How did such a finite killer become so damned infamous? Because it comes directly from estrogen injections given to animals that are bred for our consumption. Why do you think Europe won't accept any of our meats as imports? Have no doubts about it. Did you know that women who receive too many hormones from medication also develop breast cancer? Several birth control pills have been recalled for this reason alone. In the years 2010 and 2011, more than two hundred thousand females were diagnosed with breast cancer, and forty thousand of them died each year.

The Four Scariest Facts

1 Every three minutes a woman in the U.S. is diagnosed with breast cancer.

2 Breast cancer is the leading cancer among women.

3 Eighty five percent of women with breast cancer have no family history of the disease. (Don't let them tell you it is hereditary, that's just their cover-up).

4 Changes in certain genes (BRCA1 and BRCA2) make women more susceptible.

So when did breast cancer become so prevalent? When did the number of women with breast cancer increase at such alarming rates? Was it when corporations starting paying farmers with big feed lots extra money for injecting estrogen (a female growth hormone) into turkeys, chickens, pigs and cows? Well of course! The animals grow larger and have more meat on their bones, so more meat equals more money.

Excess hormones cause tumors to form, and tumors that aren't caught early spread to the rest of the body. Have no doubts, young females getting breast cancer when as young as ten years old means those girls are getting hormones boosted to a level so high that tumors are created in the breasts to try to contain them. Women, this is happening to you and your female children right now. This is not a bunch of hype. Stop eating artificial sweeteners and toxic meat. And boys over-indulging in fast food are likely to be the men who end up with prostate cancer.

I watched a special on CNN about a link between breast cancer and red meat. I got hopeful, because I thought they would really come out with the hard truth. Then at the end of the brief segment, they ruined the whole thing by acting naïve about why red meat could possibly cause breast cancer? They mentioned estrogen and animals for a second, and then moved on. I wonder how breast cancer and red meat could possibly be linked? Give me a break.

Lymph Nodes and deodorant

To understand breast cancer requires an understanding about the importance and function of the female lymph system. Believe it or not, trying to beat back body odor may be making some women sick.

So, what is a lymph node, and why should I care?

The word lymph describes a clear whitish/yellowish fluid that contains white blood cells, proteins, and some red blood cells. The lymphatic system is an essential part of the immune system, which helps the body fight infections or cancers. Because breast cancer often spreads first to the auxiliary (underarm) lymph nodes from the breast, determining whether the lymph nodes contain cancer is an essential part of the breast cancer diagnostic process. The status of the lymph nodes helps physicians determine the stage of breast cancer, and in turn, determine proper treatment. The lymphatic system consists of a network of vessels that drain tissue fluid (lymph) into lymph nodes, larger fluid-containing lymph ducts, and specialized organs involved in the immune system. The lymph nodes and organs act as a type of filter, removing invading organisms and abnormal cells from the lymph fluid, therefore processing them in a way that allows the body to fight these harmful agents.

The bean-shaped lymph nodes of the lymphatic system are connected by vessels. Lymph nodes are usually present in clusters in the armpits, on either side of the neck, and in the groin. The lymph nodes filter lymph fluid and trap foreign materials. Any fluid absorbed by the lymphatic system passes through at least one lymph node before it returns to circulation. The lymph nodes may become enlarged or swollen when they fight an infection since they must produce additional white blood cells. They may feel tender or inflamed as they are actively fighting a foreign body. Sometimes, the lymphatic vessels will become visible as thin red lines along a limb as the result of an infection. Lymph nodes may also swell from the formation of an abscess/tumor in the nodes or if they contain cancer cells.

Why is aluminum in deodorant? Trash that breast cancer causing product right now!

Antiperspirant, as the name reveals, prevents you from perspiring, thus preventing the body from purging toxins from below the armpits. These toxins remain in your system, and the body deposits them in the lymph nodes below the arms, since it can't sweat them out. This causes a high concentration of toxins that leads to cell mutation (cancer).

Nearly all breast cancer tumors occur in the upper outside quadrant of the breast area, which is where the lymph nodes are located. Most commercial brands of antiperspirants and deodorants contain aluminum chlorohydrate or aluminum zirconium. These compounds are readily absorbed by the body, and the aluminum portion of the molecule ionizes, forming free radical aluminum. This passes freely across cell membranes and forms a physical plug, that when dissolved is selectively absorbed by the liver, kidney, brain, cartilage and bone marrow. It is this concentration of aluminum that has been the source for concern in the medical community, and has prompted the research being done on Alzheimer's disease and breast cancer victims. Try *Adidas* no-aluminum deodorant for woman. It's one big step in the right direction. Thanks Adidas!

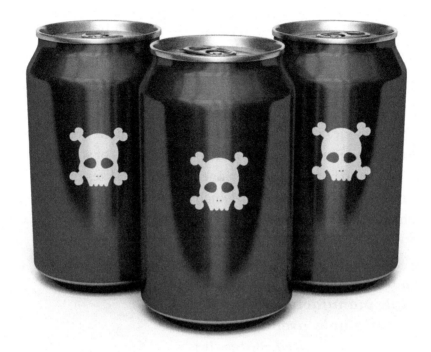

Chapter 19
Soft Drinks

Soda that is consumed on a regular basis, whether diet or sugar-loaded soda, has a major impact on your health and happiness. Over time, you will suffer consequences, so begin your education of its cumulative effects now and know what to avoid. *Most school hallways are lined with vending machines that sell soft drinks.* It's not uncommon for schools to make marketing deals with leading soft drink companies from which they receive commissions—based on a percentage of sales at each school—and sometimes a lump-sum payment.

The revenues are used for various academic and after-school activities, but what activity could be worth devastating the students' health, which is exactly what consuming all that soda is doing? Getting rid of vending machines in schools—or replacing their contents with pure water and healthy snacks—could make a big difference." Grades slipping? Can't concentrate? Are you tired after lunch every day? Wonder why? Sugar crash!

So, what's in that fancy can or plastic bottle that gets kids so buzzed?

Phosphoric Acid: This acid may interfere with the body's ability to use calcium, which can lead to osteoporosis or softening of the teeth and bones. Phosphoric acid also neutralizes the hydrochloric acid in your stomach, which can interfere with digestion, making it difficult to utilize nutrients.

Sugar (high fructose corn syrup is a GMO chemical concoction): *Soft drink manufacturers are the largest single user of refined sugar in the United States.* It is a proven fact that sugar increases insulin levels, which can lead to high blood pressure, high cholesterol, heart disease, diabetes, weight gain, premature aging and many more negative side effects. Most sodas include over one hundred percent of the RDA of sugar. And you guessed it, they use the white, bleached sugar, not to mention pesticide GMO corn breeding.

Aspartame: This is the worst chemical ever approved in the history of foods. This chemical is used as a sugar substitute in diet soda. There are over ninety two health side effects associated with aspartame consumption, including brain tumors, birth defects, diabetes, emotional disorders and epileptic seizures. When aspartame is stored for long periods of time or kept in warm areas it changes to methanol, an alcohol that converts to formaldehyde and formic acid, which are known carcinogens.

Caffeine: Caffeinated drinks cause jitters, insomnia, high blood pressure, irregular heartbeat, elevated blood cholesterol levels, vitamin and mineral depletion, breast lumps, birth defects, and perhaps some forms of cancer. I'm not saying get rid of it all, just watch how much you take in daily, that's all.

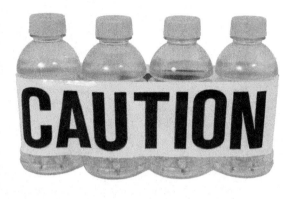

Tap Water: Straight tap water, like from your kitchen sink, tub or shower can carry any number of chemicals including fluoride, chlorine, lead, cadmium, and various organic pollutants. Tap water is the main ingredient in bottled soft drinks. Chlorine is the number one cancer contributor. Consuming fluoride, chlorine, lead, and cadmium regularly leads to cancer, bone loss and Alzheimer's disease. Only drink water that is either natural spring water or has been put through *reverse osmosis.* If you can afford it, get a filtration system for your whole house.

Soda is one of the main reasons, nutritionally speaking, why many people suffer health problems. Aside from the negative effects of the soda itself, drinking a lot of soda is likely to leave you with little appetite for vegetables, protein and other food that your body needs. If you are still drinking soda, stopping the habit is an easy way to improve your health. Pure water is a much better choice. If you must drink a carbonated beverage, try sparkling mineral water. There's nothing like it. You'll love it. The chemical war is on everyday. Defend yourself. Shield your body.

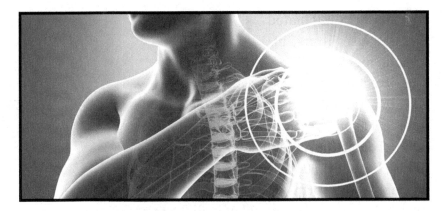

Chapter 20
Fibromyalgia

Fibromyalgia is a disorder that currently affects over five million Americans. It is a condition characterized by chronic muscle pain, irritable bowel syndrome, sleep disorders, anxiety and fatigue. Since the cause is not understood, several medications are available for managing symptoms, including analgesics and antidepressants. Conventional medicine mainly treats and suppresses symptoms using pharmaceuticals rather than looking for root causes of illnesses and disorders.

To the contrary, in Europe, where doctors get bonuses for actually healing their patients and curing them of diseases and disorders, attacking the front end of a problem is the first order of business.

Could it be that the body's inability to process, utilize, and excrete these unnatural products, which are approved by the FDA, is the main cause of fibromyalgia? Some *wild guesses* at the cause include stress injuries and psychological trauma, or even post-surgery stress. If any of these prove true, then this is the time when the human body needs nutrients the most.

One suspected culprit behind fibromyalgia is gluten, a key ingredient for giving many foods their chewy-ness and adding bulk to packaged food products. Gluten is everywhere in American grocery stores, including bread, pasta, cakes, oatmeal, salad dressings, and even canned soup. Gluten can interfere with absorption of vital nutrients and cause skin rashes, arthritis, and intense abdominal pain. Huge pharmaceutical companies are making money from this "epidemic style" disorder. And why are four out of five cases of fibromyalgia females. Aren't women consuming more of the diet foods than men?

According to a study by the Annals of Pharmacotherapy, the use of aspartame increases pain for people who have fibromyalgia. Women who decreased their intake of aspartame and MSG (monosodium glutamate) experienced decreases in pain, and then, when the additives were introduced back into their diet, the pain levels increased immediately.

Jump start the healing process by eliminating "excito-toxins," or poisons, from the diet. Many chemical food agents and additives lead to neurotoxicity when used in excess, especially when consumed on an empty stomach. Neurotoxicity is an umbrella term which covers nearly every single symptom listed under fibromyalgia. Think about it. If you look into natural remedies for this, you will find all the answers. Natural remedies may include using magnesium, vitamin D, and natural supplements that boost dopamine and serotonin levels. Vitamin B complex is important for balancing the central nervous system. Look into herbs as natural remedies also. Passion flower helps with stress and anxiety. Licorice (root powder) aids in digestion. Milk thistle, dandelion and reishi mushroom are excellent for cleansing organs like the liver and kidneys, and also for boosting immunity. Get out of the "dark" and into the light. The answer is in WHAT you eat.

In other words, cover your nutritional needs first and always remember, "Let thy food be thy medicine and thy medicine be thy food." —Hippocrates.

http://www.naturalnews.com/033874_fibromyalgia_causes.html#ixzz2lTgVCreQ

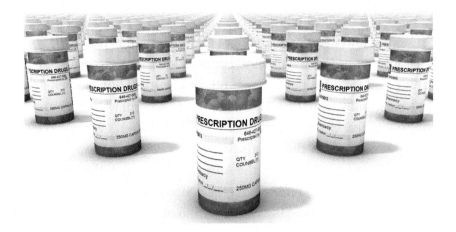

Chapter 21
Medicine Cabinet

Have a loss of energy? Have a loss of drive? Not sure why? Your headaches and sore throats aren't going away fast enough? Did you hear? A whole boatload of over-the-counter cold and flu meds has been recalled. Check your med cabinet. Google them all and check the ingredients. Trust me. They'll take away your happiness later on. They'll kill your momentum. You won't get well soon enough. Finish reading this book and take another look at the cures. There are all kinds of natural cures for what America calls disease and symptoms of those chronic ailments.

The evil twins sucralose and aspartame are found in lots of medicine too! Some doctors prescribe medications that contain aspartame for IBS. Plus, sinus meds lead to infections, like nasal and bronchial by shrinking membranes and preventing normal drainage and suppressing productive coughing. Oh, you didn't know?

American doctors push them on us like they're vitamins. Just say no! And so to conclude, the cumulative effect is usually first noticed when your organs begin to malfunction or fail, or

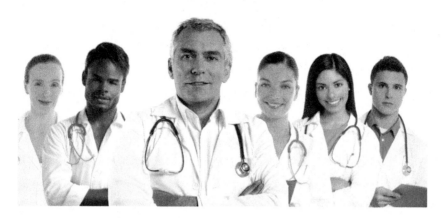

when they develop tumors that show up on x-rays or impede other normal body functions. But you can't live without your kidneys, or your liver, and unfortunately, those are the first to go.

Your liver plays a major role in metabolism and has a number of functions in the body including glycogen storage, plasma protein synthesis, and drug detoxification. This organ also is the largest gland in the human body. It produces bile, which is important in digestion. It performs and regulates a wide variety of high-volume biochemical reactions requiring specialized tissues. 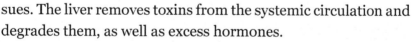 The liver removes toxins from the systemic circulation and degrades them, as well as excess hormones.

Your kidneys are organs functioning to maintain proper water and electrolyte balance, regulate acid-base concentration, and filter the blood of metabolic wastes, which are then excreted as urine. They excrete waste products produced by metabolism, including the nitrogenous wastes.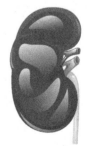

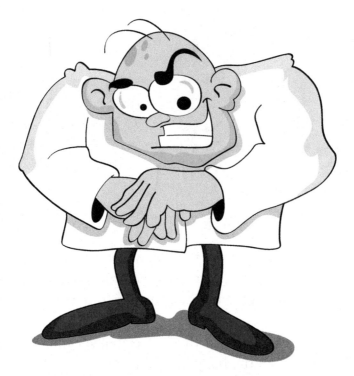

Chapter 22
Side Effects

Western Medicine's approach—is that we begin searching for the cure for something after it has completely developed into a serious condition. ***Then we over-prescribe and the drugs under-deliver.*** After that, we get sent home, yeah, that's right, with doctors saying things like everything's "going to be fine, just stay low stress and stay on the medication you're given, and everything's going to be just fine.

Then comes the relapse ...

"Go home and get some sleep," they always say! That serious condition you had before has been "completely addressed." But really, it's been covered up with drugs that give you minor side effects, meanwhile, your body recovers temporarily, only to fall inevitably into a massive relapse, and that's when they pull you back into the hospital, and you're laid out in a bed thinking "déjà vu."

Then it sinks in, that maybe the drugs just covered up the symptoms of the attack, while the problem just spread, and you thought that those migraine headaches, sudden loss of vision, and dry mouth were just the tail end of dealing with this whole horrible thing. Suddenly one night at the quiet hospital, laid out in the blue bed, being waited on hand and foot, watching bad T.V., probably going to the bathroom in that nasty little pan, you start thinking deeper, maybe philosophically, because it seems like these doctors and nurses and parents and friends all have the same advice, "hang in there!" It echoes in your brain, and you start trying to heal yourself mentally, but you're not sure if that's really going to work. So you start thinking.

Is it bad karma? Did I do something to deserve this, because I don't remember what it was, if I did? Does God love me? Does He even know this is happening to me? How could *He* let it happen? Or maybe you're an atheist and you're not expecting any rescue—you figure it's your time to go. So you're laying there with symptoms, side effects, bed sores, bad food, lousy service, too much television, rare visitors, and you're just going to "Take the strikes as they come?!"

Sorry, that's not my ticket. That's not my style. I don't like feeling sick and not being able to do God's business. The human body is fragile and vulnerable. I take care of mine and I am a defensive consumer, so I can avoid accidents. Won't you please join me as I avoid and dispel the ridiculous "too-little, too-late philosophy. Don't poison your soul. The new cure for cancer is under construction. I've dug up the truth and exposed it, now you can use it to live longer. Sometimes, the drugs used in cancer treatment appear to be as harmful to healthy tissue as to the cancer itself, according to newly reported cellular and animal studies, which explain the poorly understood condition known as chemo brain. *Avoid the side effects of late treatment, and treat yourself to a long, healthy life.* Side effects are the after affects of a consumer market that ignorantly consumes chemicals.

Have you heard the side effects at the end of the latest new drug commercials? It's ridiculous that they are allowed on the market.

Decrease in vision (Viagra)—What does that mean? ... Okay, so one sunny day, all of a sudden all you can see is shadows? That sounds really safe—and worth the risk too. Wait, what was my problem again ... I can't remember, someone flip on a light!

Anal leakage (aspartame): That is my favorite! So you're not fat anymore, but your rear end leaks fluid all day that looks like used oil from an old pickup truck. Not pretty!

Nausea—Oh, this is a good one. Hey, whatever problem the medicine is clearing up for me, I guarantee you I won't be able to appreciate it while I feel like vomiting all day.

Increased blood pressure—oh cool ... so my problem is clearing up, but I better not get excited about it, or I may have a heart attack. Can I *supersize* that please, with some internal bleeding?

Depression—perfect! I'll be in a real good mood when my condition clears up. Why not just tell us the side effect is feeling like suicide.

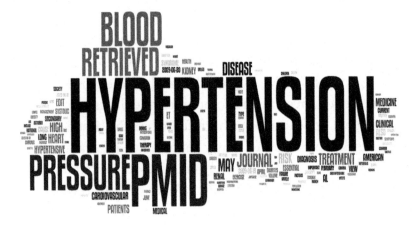

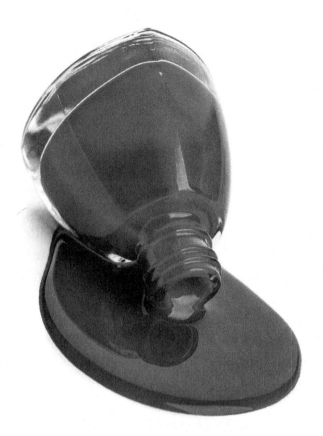

Chapter 23
Nail Polish

It's nice when a woman knows how to use makeup tastefully. It would also be nice to know she's using makeup that doesn't have chemicals in it, so after twenty years go by, she's not getting some of those "beauty spots" surgically removed from her face by the dermatologist. That's when you might want to know what dibutyl phthalate DBP is and what it does to your body. DBP is a chemical used to keep nail polish from chipping, and it has been connected to cancer in lab animals, as well as long-term fertility issues in newborns, leaving the cosmetics industry in a heavy debate over whether to continue use of the ingredient. The sad part is there are few regulations on ingredients in cosmetics in the U.S.

You would be hard pressed to find any, so trust me on this.

Environmental groups are calling for a ban on DBP in the United States, and some big name companies such as *Estee Lauder* have removed the chemical from their products, which tells you something is seriously wrong with it, but still other brands continue to use it. Hey, money's money, right? Remember, when they say it's "not about the money," it always is.

While the FDA must approve nail polishes before they can be sold, of course there are no laws that require companies to prove their products are safe first, so what does it matter? Products are usually only tested for acute and immediate reactions before they are put on the market. And so continue the spoils of a rotten system. Contrary to popular belief, industrial chemicals in consumer products are essentially unregulated in the United States, except for chemicals added directly to food, there is no legal requirement for health and safety testing or human exposure monitoring for any chemical in commerce. The same chemicals, ironically, are often tightly regulated as pollutants. Go figure! Long-term health concerns such as cancer or reproductive toxicity are rarely, if ever, tested.

The FDA says they have no legal authority to regulate products and keep companies from including chemicals in cosmetics. *Oh yeah, then create a subsidiary agency, you jerks!* A September 2000 study by the U.S. Centers for Disease Control and Prevention reported that there was DBP in every person they tested, with the highest levels detected in women aged twenty to forty. The CDC had a scientific guess that the exposure might be from cosmetics, although people can also come into contact with DBP from vinyl shower curtains or children's plastic toys.

DBP is just one ingredient in a melting pot of pollutants that contaminate every person in the industrialized world. Everyone in the United States carries more than one hundred chemical pollutants, pesticides, and toxic metals in their body. To test one hundred chemicals in combinations of three for just one health

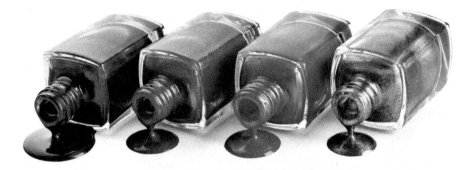

effect, say, um, cancer, for example, as opposed to birth defects, would require over one hundred thousand new tests. There are currently more than seventy five thousand chemicals licensed for use in the United States. At least fifteen thousand are sold in volumes greater than ten thousand pounds per year! Under the Toxic Substances Control Act the EPA has regulated just five chemicals.

One report entitled *Not Too Pretty* cited an independent lab that found at least one type of phthalate in face creams, lotions, shampoos, hairsprays, deodorants and fragrances. *Campaign for Safe Cosmetics* calls for nail polish manufactures to remove DBP from their products, and sign a pledge to not use chemicals that are known or—strongly suspected of causing cancer, mutation or birth defects in their products, and for them to implement substitution plans that replace hazardous materials with safer alternatives in every single market they serve. DBP is a horror story come to life! This carcinogenic, gender-bending, toxic chemical DBP causes a number of birth defects in lab animals, primarily to male offspring, including testicular atrophy, a reduced sperm count, and defects in the structure of the penis. "Hey Honey, Junior doesn't seem too happy with this weird side effect that my make-up handed down to him."

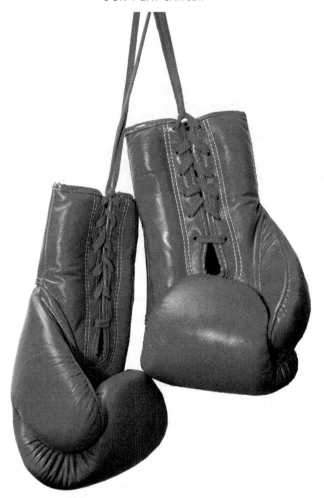

Chapter 24
Fight back!

A few years ago I decided enough was enough, and I changed my eating habits almost entirely, within one year. It's not that my eating habits were so bad to begin with, but I was *cheating* in more realms than I realized, and it all got pointed out to me, over time. The more I studied, the more I realized I wasn't practicing what I was preaching. I had stopped eating meat and had cut out most dairy. I rarely ate sweets, but I ate a lot of chips, mayonnaise on sandwiches, and I was still cooking a lot of food in processed oils at high heat. I found out also that I was eating a lot of dead foods – meaning foods that were baked, fried, grilled, broiled, boiled, barbecued or steamed way too long. I was cooking my food to death. I didn't know a thing about "live" food, except that salad was good for you. What a wake-up call I received, over and over, when I woke up feeling lethargic, or just couldn't seem to get anything done at the gym or jogging. When you realize the total amount of GMO food that you are eating, and you realize you are supposed to be eating at least seventy percent of your food whole or raw, that's when you know about energy, positivity, immunity and health and happiness.

Don't let history repeat itself – stay informed!

Nearly one hundred years ago, the American Medical Association (AMA) began removing nutritional education from medical schools in America. Medical doctors would no longer understand anything about using food as medicine (or be allowed to suggest it), and all mid-wives, Native American herbalists and natural healers would be referred to in medical journals as "quacks." The Western Medicine philosophy would soon come to be that no food in the world could ever heal a human being or cure any disease or disorder. In fact, only pharmaceuticals and vaccines would ever be able to make that claim and get away with it, whether in peer reviews, medical and science journals, scientific studies or labeled as such on products.

At the current time, it is illegal for any food, herb, tincture or superfood product to say that it cures anything, yet medications advertised on TV since 1997 can say they treat all kinds of diseases and disorders, even though the side effects are horrendous, some of the time including internal bleeding, blindness, deafness and even suicide.

Mother Nature, on the other hand, has a cure for everything and also offers prevention and immunity for everything under the sun. Nutritionists and naturopathic physicians will tell you all day that organic fruits and organic vegetables are the key to healing and living a healthy life. A plant-based diet can heal nearly any health problem, and the body is like a machine that fires on all cylinders when given the correct fuel. Take this knowledge and be on your way to health freedom and natural living, where you have lots of energy, rarely ever get sick, can think critically all the time, can be spiritual and independent and take care of your family! Learn and grow from it. Don't eat cancer. Don't drink cancer. Be organic.

Read labels. Read professional articles regarding the foods you eat regularly. Do the research ahead of time. If you are in doubt, throw it out! You don't have to finish something you bought just because it's already paid for. You can benefit your body by getting rid of it and finding organic. The price is a tradeoff in the long run and your body rewards you in the short term! You see. It works.

Fighting back means standing up for what is right. Whole food is right. Spring water is right. Natural remedies are right. Being a defensive consumer keeps you ready for anything, like a good mixed martial artist. Don't fall for Big Food's food tricks that slow you down, dampen your thinking, pull from your positive outlook, or just rain on your parade. This is your life so live it safely and with prudence.

The smart phone app *Fooducate* could be the beginning of the end for GMO. You see, one of the biggest obstacles holding people back from eating healthy is easy access to *resourceful information*, about chemicals in foods, or natural remedies and supplements, and about new choices to make right at the store. If only technology made something for your phone, so you could scan every product's barcode

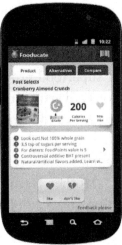

and get a quick, reliable summary of what you're really getting. For instance, is it GMO? Does it contain gluten? Am I allergic to the ingredients? Guess what? The smart phone app already exists, and has been around for a few years, but hardly anyone knows about it. That's all about to change.

http://www.fooducate.com/

Planet Earth is chock full of natural resources, foods that heal the body, herbs and mushrooms that build immunity, extracts and seed oils that cure diseases, and if no food scientists ever took any of it into a lab and cooked it with chemicals, there would be far less disease and disorder, far less obesity and cancer, and far less of a need to put a HUGE filter on everything you consider purchasing.

http://store.naturalnews.com/Superfoods_c_4.html

Not everyone has a smart phone, but millions now do. If you are not one of those fortunate owners of a smart phone, you may want to bring a friend or loved one along with you who has one, and bring them with you to every store where you buy food.

Remember the old saying, "Let your fingers do the walking?" In other words, let your fingers do the research, if you don't have the time. The smart phone app will uncover the lies, the food toxins, the food criminals, and expose them, right on the spot! If you read labels at all, you can read the *Fooducate* app even easier.

Now you don't have to try to figure out what all those long crazy words or ingredients mean that you can't even pronounce, and you will know whether they include GMOs, pesticide, insecticide, herbicide, or toxic food coloring, aluminum (heavy metals), gluten, MSG, Aspartame, or other cancer-causing, heart attack-breeding junk that's put in our "natural" food. Even organic foods can be checked for a rating, so you can make a fast judgment call as to whether or not you want the ingredients of a particular product to get past your "body guards" and enter the temple of your soul.

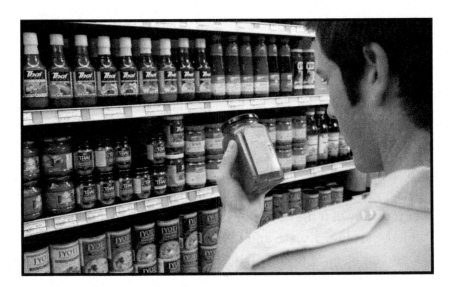

Scan the bar codes of everything you consider buying and eating!

■ Find out what is GMO or is Non-GMO in seconds!

■ Find out if something is vegan, vegetarian and organic - instantly!

■ Filter out wheat, gluten, food colorings and food allergens!

■ Get a quick calorie count and fat content (the good and bad fats)!

You should not waste time wondering what you're eating ever again, just scan the bar code, read a short description and look at the rating it gets. *Fooducate* grades (rates) foods and beverages on a scale from A to D. There are 10 distinct grades: A, A-, B+, B, B-, C+, C, C-, D+ and D. These grades are based on nutrition, ingredients, and processing (if any). *Fooducate* even accepts feedback if you disagree with their rating! How considerate is that?

http://www.fooducate.com/

It's "kill or be killed" when it comes to GMO

The best part of the *Fooducate* app is that it gives concise explanations along with a grading system developed by scientists, dietitians and concerned parents. I believe that if everyone started scanning bar codes with the *Fooducate* app and used the GMO/non-GMO indicator, there could be a wave of millions of people who avoid GMO entirely in the near future, and maybe, just maybe, we could put an end to GMO altogether.

http://www.seedsofdeception.com/

Take the "die" out of your diet right now!

Get the bug killer and weed killer out of your food. Do not buy pesticide food. You can kill disease before it starts killing you. Never let it into your system in the first place. Protect your cells so they won't mutate. Basically, if you filter out GMO from every shopping experience, you will be filtering the chemicals that Big Food is putting in vegetable seeds and on the vegetables growing on the farms across the Midwest. The long-term research is in, and it is reliable and scary. Pay attention. Get the app and scan the bar codes. It's that simple. You can search for bleach, ammonia, MSG, Aspartame, and lots of other major food criminals! Fooducate is getting 5 star reviews!

Juicing and blending smoothies will extend your healthy life!

How do you live to be one hundred and ten? Tell someone you're over one hundred years old, and they might assume the worst right away, guessing that you have a dozen medication bottles next to the bed and that your health is quickly deteriorating. How could it be that a man who's going on one hundred and eleven, and taking no medication, who simply eats fresh vegetables, olive oil, honey, cinnamon, garlic and chocolate, can bounce around his kitchen like he's half his age?

When Bernando LaPallo of Mesa, Arizona tells his secrets of longevity and vitality, your jaw drops to the ground, wondering how he avoided Alzheimer's, brittle bones, cancer and diabetes. Could it be that Western Medicine has it all wrong, and all we ever needed were raw veggies, super-foods, raw nuts and berries, and some barley soup? Maybe Medicare and Medicaid should broker a deal with the makers of power juicers and call it "Universal Healthcare."

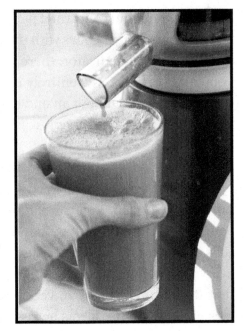

The Fountain of Youth is Organic and Raw

Here's the fountain of youth "natural remedies" you can turn into your own daily regimen, so your mind, body, and spirit can thrive well into triple digits:

- High quality, organic, cold-pressed extra virgin olive oil: use on the skin as lotion; use as salad dressing; known to lessen risks of colon cancer and heart disease.
- Dark, organic chocolate: reduces stress; helps with depression; lowers blood pressure and cholesterol levels.
- Organic garlic: helps fight coughs and colds; considered nature's antibiotic; helps with digestion and intestinal problems.
- Organic cinnamon: antibacterial and antifungal; reduces proliferation of leukemia and lymphoma cancer cells.
- Organic honey: helps you lose weight; nature's energy booster; has antioxidant and antibacterial properties.
- Juice organic raw vegetables: A decent juicer costs less than $100.

And if you're not familiar with this style of turning fresh "veggies" into a drink, try these surprisingly tasty combinations with your new juicer: Carrot, cucumber, sweet potato, a quarter size slice of fresh ginger, and freshly squeezed lime. Also try this: celery, kale, Granny Smith apple for sweetness, and of course lemon or lime juice. Plus you don't have to let the vegetable pulp go to waste. Use it to enhance flavors in dishes or to bulk up your stew, or mix it with quinoa and maybe some diced onions as an accent.

Nature provides the untainted answer to building a strong vascular and immune system - one that can fight off infection, stress, arthritis, and even stave off the aging process. If you have not already, do further research into foods which are rich in antioxidants, enzymes, phyto-nutrients, and be sure to research foods that detoxify your body and destroy free radicals.

http://www.naturalnews.com/034666_longevity_aging_prevention.html#ixzz2q25Qa0ql

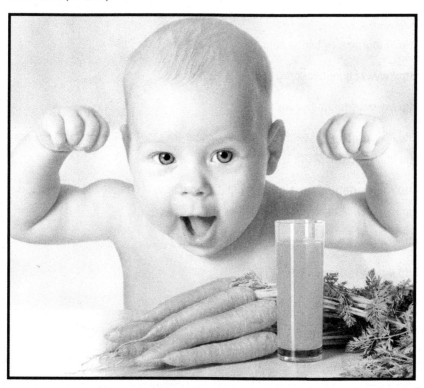

Sources

http://www.thelancet.com/journals/lancet/iss

http://www.naturalnews.com/033568_obesity_America.html#ixzz2pRYED9O2

http://www.naturalnews.com/034483_fried_foods_health_damage.html#ixzz2pRVm0H4S

http://breathing.com/articles/canola-oil.htm

http://www.naturalnews.com/038670_heavy_metals_chelation_foods.html#ixzz2ppzkymzZ

http://labs.naturalnews.com/Video-Food-Science-Breakthrough-Announcements.html

http://www.naturalnews.com/041140_addiction_brain_chemistry_mental_health.html#ixzz2pRWn0bf5

http://www.alternatives-for-alcoholism.com/about.html

http://programs.webseed.com

http://www.cbgnetwork.org

http://www.drfuhrman.com

http://www.naturalnews.com/043202_cancer_health_basics_disease_prevention.html#ixzz2pRe84GIh

http://www.naturalnews.com/042336_processed_foods_dead_nutrients_organic_produce.html#ixzz2pRf013XD

http://www.consumerreports.org/cro/pork0113.htm

http://www.foxnews.com

http://www.naturalnews.com/superbugs.html

http://www.naturalnews.com/038335_pork_superbugs_bacteria.html#ixzz2pN3NQr5V

http://www.naturalnews.com/028105_Fibroids_remedies.html#ixzz2pN3bhr2i

http://www.nongmoproject.org

http://www.fooducate.com

http://www.naturalnews.com/041302_toxic_foods_symptoms_msg_headache.
html#ixzz2pRiL633W

http://dev.www.health.harvard.edu/healthbeat/HB_web/getting-out-the-gluten.
htm

http://www.naturalnews.com/042045_food_labels_demystified_certified_organic.html#ixzz2pRoglnAa

http://www.naturalnews.com/038170_gluten_sensitivity_symptoms_intolerance.html#ixzz2pRp5JFVp

http://holisticprimarycare.net

http://www.organic.org/home/faq

http://organicfood.einnews.com

http://www.naturalnews.com/037992_organic_food_gmo.html#ixzz2pRzDVN63

http://www.naturalnews.com/034101_microwaveable_containers_plastics.
html#ixzz2pMm4Gxoh

http://www.naturalnews.com/030651_microwave_cooking_cancer.html

http://www.naturalnews.com/023011_microwave_food_oven.
html#ixzz2pMnORTYM

http://www.naturalnews.com/028438_beef_hormones.html#ixzz2pN42hUxQ

http://www.naturalnews.com/019557_artificial_hormones_red_meat.
html#ixzz2pN26REJm

http://www.naturalnews.com/022913_rBGH_milk_cows.html#ixzz2pN2lFecL

http://www.naturalnews.com/038335_pork_superbugs_bacteria.
html#ixzz2pN3HAoGG

http://www.naturalnews.com/040807_GM_salmon_franken-fish_genetic_pollution.html#ixzz2pfEXY2Qu

http://www.naturalnews.com/040980_big_food_toxic_ingredients_diet_warning.html#ixzz2pN6ImiKY

http://www.ers.usda.gov/Data/BiotechCrops/

http://news.bbc.co.uk/2/hi/health/3586573.st...

http://www.naturalnews.com/034209_GMOs_questions.html#ixzz2pRdq6rUL

http://www.naturalnews.com/042830_vegetarians_restaurants_eating_dead_animals.html#ixzz2pRvzHkHL

http://www.thedailygreen.com

http://www.rawfullytempting.com

http://www.peopleforanimalsindia.org

http://www.v1.thehealingjournal.com

http://www.naturalnews.com/042688_natural_medicine_cancer_cures_government_agencies.html#ixzz2jENDDz4t

Evolution vs. Neanderthal; *The Moral Animal* by Robert Wright

Thick Face, Black Heart

Cancer Prevention Coalition

Information that Empowers

Carcinogens: Free Encyclopedia

Clemson Extension: Home and Garden Information Center

Chemicals and Foods

Hormonal Growth Accelerants

New Zealand Food Safety Authority

Organic Consumers Association: Processed Meats Cause Cancer

Mission Possible International: New Cancer Study 2006

Aspartamekills.com

Colette Chuda Environmental Fund

Sucralose Kills: The Rat that Told Humans What Not to Eat.

Futurepundit.com: Archives on Sequences with Mice, Rats. 2006

Medical News Today: Aspartame Causes Cancer in Rats. Still approved for humans.

Diabetes Monitor.com

Cancer.Org: Cancer Projections/Death Rates.

Microwave Ovens and Death.

Child Life: Health World Online

Campaign for Safe Cosmetics

Jane Russell's Health Facts

Natural News; the best health news available 24/7 on line

Acknowledgments

Special thanks to my Mother. She and I have had discussions late at night for years, drinking tea and talking about life and how to live it longer and healthier. Thanks Mom for all your help and guidance. I love you. Those times are priceless to me. Thanks internet: You made it easy for a guy with a master's degree to find relevant information, resources, and reliable nutritionists, like Mike Adams and David Wolfe. And thanks to my creative writing instructor from college, Dr. Coleman Barks, for his inspiration. Lastly, thanks to Köehler Books for recognizing this work and publishing it so I can get this message out to the world!